Keto Cookbook and keto Bread for Women

3 Books in 1

The Complete Guide For All Women To Lose Weight and Shaper Their Body With delicious Low-Carb Recipes and Learn On How to Make a Special Keto Bread

By

Sofia Wilson

© Copyright 2021 - All rights reserved.

The following Book is reproduced below with the goal of providing information that is as accurate and reliable as possible. Regardless, purchasing this Book can be seen as consent to the fact that both the publisher and the author of this book are in no way experts on the topics discussed within and that any recommendations or suggestions that are made herein are for entertainment purposes only. Professionals should be consulted as needed prior to undertaking any of the action endorsed herein.

This declaration is deemed fair and valid by both the American Bar Association and the Committee of Publishers Association and is legally binding throughout the United States.

Furthermore, the transmission, duplication, or reproduction of any of the following work including specific information will be considered an illegal act irrespective of if it is done electronically or in print. This extends to creating a secondary or tertiary copy of the work or a recorded copy and is only allowed with the express written consent from the Publisher. All additional right reserved.

The information in the following pages is broadly considered a truthful and accurate account of facts and as such, any inattention, use, or misuse of the information in question by the reader will render any resulting actions solely under their purview. There are no scenarios in which the publisher or the original author of this work can be in any fashion deemed liable for any hardship or damages that may befall them after undertaking information described herein.

Additionally, the information in the following pages is intended only for informational purposes and should thus be thought of as universal. As befitting its nature, it is presented without assurance regarding its prolonged validity or interim quality. Trademarks that are mentioned are done without written consent and can in no way be considered an endorsement from the trademark holder.

Table of Contents

KETO FOR WOMEN

INTRODUCTION 10

CHAPTER 1: WHAT IS THE KETOGENIC DIET? 16

CHAPTER 2: WHAT ARE KETONES? 21

CHAPTER 3: WHAT HAPPENS TO YOUR BODY WHEN YOU GO KETO? ... 26
Differences Between Ketosis And Ketoacidosis 26
Benefits Of Ketosis 26
Risks Of Ketosis 28

CHAPTER 4: HEAL YOUR BODY 30

CHAPTER 5: IS KETO FOR YOU? 35

CHAPTER 6: BENEFITS OF KETOGENIC DIET FOR WOMEN 38

CHAPTER 7: USING KETO DIET TO CONTROL OR PREVENT AGE-RELATED CONDITIONS 41

CHAPTER 8: SUPPORTING BASIC BODY SYSTEMS 45

CHAPTER 9: DIABETES PREVENTION 48
What Is Diabetes? 48
Types Of Diabetes 48
Is The Keto Diet Suitable For People With Diabetes? 51
Can The Keto Diet Prevent Diabetes? 51

CHAPTER 10: DIETARY EXCHANGE THROUGH THE MENSTRUAL CYCLE 53

CHAPTER 11: KETOGENIC DIET AND FERTILITY 57

CHAPTER 12: BASIC RECIPES 63
Keto Tortillas With Linseed 66
Keto Tortilla With Almond Flour And Coconut 67
EMPANADAS OF KETO MEAT 68
Keto Pizza 69
Keto Cream Of Mushrooms With Spinach 71

CHAPTER 13: FOOD CHOICE 73

CHAPTER 14: BREAKFAST 78
Cups Of Egg, Ham, And Cheese 80
Stuffed Peppers 81

CHAPTER 15: LUNCH 83
Cobb Egg Salad 84
Stuffed Avocados 86
Keto Bacon Sushi 88

CHAPTER 16: DINNERS 90
Breasts Stuffed With Pesto Sauce And Mozzarella Cheese 92
Hake With Romesco Sauce And Vegetables 93
Broccoli And Sausage Tortilla 94

CHAPTER 17: SWEET TOOTHS, SNACKS AND DESSERTS 96
Eggplant French Fries 98
Bacon And Cheddar Cheese Balls 99
Spinach, Artichoke And Cream Cheese Dip 99
Focaccia Bread With Garlic And Rosemary 100
Mexican-Style Sausages 101
Lettuce Cubes With Prickly Pear Salad 101
Prepared Olives 102
Cauliflower Bits With Peanut Butter 102
Chard Skewers With Ham And Cheese 103
Crackers Of Crunchy Seeds And Oats 105

CHAPTER 18: KETO DRINKS 106
Keto Smoothie Chocolate 107
Smoothie For Breakfast 108

CHAPTER 19: 7 DAY MEAL PLAN: 115
Monday 115
Tuesday 115
Wednesday 115
Thursday 116
Friday 116
Saturday 116
Sunday 117

CONCLUSION 119

KETO DIET

Introduction 122

UNDERSTANDING THE KETOGENIC DIET 123
1.1 What is Keto? 123
1.2 What is the Keto diet, and how does it work? 126

BREAKFAST, LUNCH AND DINNER RECIPES 130
1 Hot Chocolate 130
2 Classic bacon with eggs 132
3 keto breakfast 134
4 Spinach and scrambled eggs 136
5 Oven pancake 137
6 Pulled Pork 140
7 Bacon Egg Cups 142
8 Granola Clusters 144
9 Crustless Quiche 146
10 Fluffy Eggs 148

11 KETO PANCAKES	150
12 FRITTATA MUFFINS	152
13 BACON OMELET	154
14 BRIE FRITTATA	155
15 FRIED RICE	157
16 THAI SOUP	160
17 BUFFALO SOUP	161
18 JALAPENO SOUP	164
19 SAUSAGE WITH PEPPERS	166
20 BEEF BARBACOA	168
21 CAULIFLOWER SHRIMP	170
22 CHEESE SPINACH	172
23 TANGY CHICKEN DRUMETTES	174
24 RANCH CHICKEN	176
25 GARLIC CHICKEN WINGS	178
26 STEAK SALAD	180
27 CATFISH	182
28 SALAD- SWEDISH STYLE	184
29 FISH MEDLEY	186
30 HAM WRAPS	188
31 ALASKAN COD	190
32 PAPRIKA OMELET	192
33 BOILED EGGS	194
34 STUFFED PEPPERS	196
35 KALE BAKE	198
36 CHEESE MEATBALLS	199
37 ITALIAN CRISPS	202
38 SPICY MEATBALLS	204
39 CHEESE STUFFED MUSHROOMS	205
40 BEEF WITH HERBS	208
41 CHINESE BEEF SKILLET	210
42 BEEF STROGANOFF	212
43 CHICKEN ZOODLES	214
44 CREAMY TUSCAN CHICKEN	216
45 TURKEY AND PEPPERS	217
46 BUTTER CHICKEN	220
47 ASPARAGUS CHICKEN	222
48 CHICKEN CHILI	224
49 TACO AVOCADOS	226
50 BROCCOLI BEEF BOWLS	228
51 CAULIFLOWER-BACON CHEESE MASH	231
52 SPAGHETTI SQUASH WITH BLUE CHEESE AND BACON	233
53 RANCH CAULIFLOWER CRACKERS	235
54 EASY CAULIFLOWER CASSEROLE	237
55 WHITE CHICKEN CHILI	239
CONCLUSION	**242**

ESSENTIAL KETO BREAD

INTRODUCTION **248**
UNDERSTANDING THE KETOGENIC DIET **249**
   1.1 WHAT IS KETO? 249
   1.2 WHAT IS THE KETO DIET, AND HOW DOES IT WORK? 252
KETO BREAD RECIPES **256**
   1 EMPANADAS 256
   2 KETO BAGELS 258
   3 HOT DOG BUNS 260
   4 CORNBREAD 262
   5 QUICK STYLE BREAD 264
   6 MEDITERRANEAN BREAD 266
   7 PARMESAN CROUTONS 268
   8 CLOUD BREAD 270
   9 GARLIC FOCACCIA 272
   10 PARMESAN CHIPS 274
   11 LOW-CARB BREAD 276
   12 PIZZA CRUST 278
   13 ZUCCHINI CIABATTA 280
   14 KETO DOSA 282
   15 SIMPLE KETO BREAD 284
   16 SEED CRACKERS 286
   17 SESAME BREAD 288
   18 HOLIDAY BREAD 290
   19 BUTTER BREAD 292
   20 BREAD TWISTS 294
   21 FRENCH TOAST 296
   22 SOFT TORTILLAS 298
   23 NUT-FREE BREAD 300
   24 FLUFFY BREAD 302
   25 90 SECONDS BREAD 304
   26 ALMOND FLOUR BREAD 306
   27 PLAIN BREAD 308
   28 FATHEAD BREAD 310
   29 BREAD ROLLS 312
   30 SIMPLE AND EASY BREAD 314
   31 GLUTEN-FREE BREAD 316
   32 COLLAGEN BREAD 318
   33 COCONUT BREAD 320
   34 MACADAMIA BREAD 322
   35 CAULIFLOWER BREAD 324
   36 KETO TORTILLAS 326
   37 BUTTERY FLATBREAD 328
   38 GLUTEN-FREE BISCUITS 330
   39 CAULIFLOWER BUNS 331

40 Low Carb Biscuits..333
41 Pizza Crust..335
42 Zucchini Bread...337
43 Blueberry Muffin Bread..339
44 Cranberry Bread 341
45 Fluffy Buns...343
46 Ultimate Buns..345
47 Dinner Rolls...347
48 Bagel Scones...349
49 Avocado bread 351
50 Croissants..353
51 Gluten-Free Bagels...355
52 Fluffy Keto Pancakes..356
53 High Protein Bread 359

CONCLUSION... 361

Keto for Women

Your Essential Guide To Living The Keto Diet With Low-Carb, High-Fat Recipes For Busy Women

By

Sofia Wilson

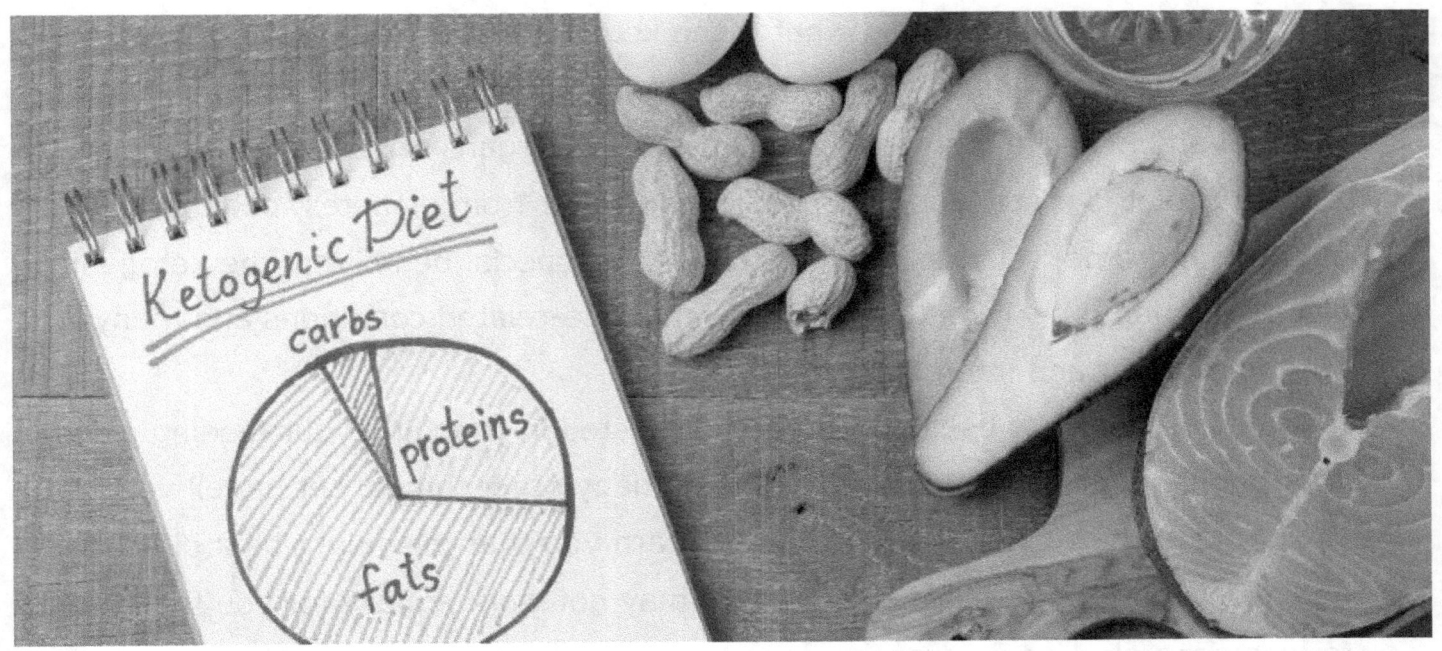

Introduction

Congratulations on purchasing Keto for women: The ultimate beginners guide to know your food needs, weight loss, diabetes prevention and boundless energy with high-fat ketogenic diet recipes and thank you for doing so.

The following chapters will provide you all the necessary information, facts and scientific explanations that you need to know and master the keto diet. You will find the details explanation on what is the keto diet based on, what are the ketones, what happens in your body when you go keto, how the ketogenic diet will heal and improve many of the processes and organs of your body, how the ketogenic diet is pretty good for people who suffer from diabetes, polycystic ovaries syndrome, seizures, and Alzheimer, the special benefits of the ketogenic diet on women, how it reduces and prevents age-related conditions and many other important and interesting information.

If you came here it is because you are interested in changing your feeding plans, your habits, your body, your lifestyle, and many other things. Let us tell you that you came to the right place. We want to warn you that this might be a difficult process, some of the things written here may not work equally for you than it did for someone else, so we want to ask you to go and see a specialist before making any change to your alimentation

There are plenty of books on this subject on the market, thanks again for choosing this one! Every effort was made to ensure it is full of as much useful information as possible, please enjoy it!

Chapter 1:
What Is The Ketogenic Diet?

The Keto or ketogenic diet consists mainly of the ingestion of 75% fats, 20% high-value biological protein and 5% low glycemic index carbohydrates. That percentage should be applied to every meal. People who want to start with this diet must understand that this is not a diet, but this is a whole new lifestyle and it should be taken as it.

We want to mention that this type of diet has years in the market and has been subject of research on many occasions, demonstrating, in all cases, the wonderful benefits it has on health. This feeding plan is not only for adults; children and teenagers could also use it; so it is highly recommended.

The Keto diet has its beginnings near the 1920s and was made specially as a treatment for the people who suffered from seizures. Over time, and after a lot of researches and studies, the diet surprisingly showed results that were really satisfactory. The first case that possibly has been registered and in which the ketogenic diet for epileptic patients was applied was in 1911. The investigation was led by two French doctors who were Gulep and Marie. They treated approximately 20 persons, between children and adults. The objective of the investigation was to apply this type of diet, added to other protocols known as intermittent fasting.

The ketogenic diet is also very popularly known to lose weight, and lower blood sugar levels considerably, but it is important to know that sugar, gluten and other components that are not within the food permitted in this diet or method of ketogenic nutrition must be eliminated.

As we mentioned above, the major part of the food that we are going to consume is healthy fats, such as avocado, bacon, and peanuts, to mention some of them. In the following chapters of this book, you will be able to see some recipes or plans that you can apply in this diet.

The objective we want to achieve applying the keto diet is to reach a metabolic state in which ketones are the primary energy source of our body. This is achieved by following the diet regularly, with commitment and discipline.

This diet is not based on dietary restrictions, but on significant changes in lifestyle and eating habits, in which we are going to eliminate from our menu processed foods based on refined flours, sugar, and soft drinks. It is a diet that manages to heal marvelously and allow adequate cellular regeneration; Therefore, it improves and even eliminates some diseases, if applied in an evaluated manner with a specialist.

And these changes in the organism are due to the fact that this feeding method gives us the adequate tools for the best functioning of the cellular environment on our organism, and it does so by providing amino acids, essential fats for our body, vitamins, and minerals. This diet is amazing since it doesn't just allow you to lose weight but also makes you feel energy levels that you haven't before.

Any diet can be ketogenic if their bases are respected and if we have the knowledge of cellular processes and metabolism. Diets that can be considered ketogenic are those that force our body to use fats as a source of energy. Fasting can be considered ketogenical since by spending so many hours without eating, the body runs out of glucose and start to use ketones instead. Known this, we can say that a diet in which the lack of carbohydrates is replaced with other foods that has high contents of nutrients can be a ketogenic diet

The main objective of the ketogenic diet is to make our body to get into ketosis, lowering or decreasing to only 5% the intake of carbohydrates. This is a diet low in carbohydrates, and rich in fats that have been compared several times with the Atkins diet and other low-carbohydrate diets, so we share the idea that any diet where these percentages of food are distributed in similar amounts are ketogenic diets, or as it is abbreviated keto diets.

When we start with the ketogenic diet, we decrease the consumption of carbohydrates and replace them with healthy fats. Once this is done, the body will reach or get into a metabolic state called ketosis. In this state, the body is going to become incredibly efficient, transforming the fats in our body into energy. This process will also convert the accumulated fat in our body into ketones, hence supplying the brain with more energy. It should be noted that this eating plan generates higher energy levels than the ones generated by the usual feeding methods.

There are some foods that should be avoided when we are implementing this diet; Some of them are the following:

- Foods with high levels of sugar such as soft drinks, candies, fruit juices, cakes (in this case we would be talking about cakes made with refined flour), and other sweets.
- Foods that are derived from wheat like rice, pasta, cereals or starches.
- Some fruits should be eliminated due to their high amount of sugars. The only fruits that will be allowed are small proportions of forest fruits such as strawberries, blackberries, kiwi.
- The vegetables or legumes. Within this classification are: sweet potatoes, carrots, cassava, among others
- Lentils, chickpeas, beans or legumes.
- Some types of sauces. We would have to evaluate their preparation, as well as the condiments to use. In the keto diet, it is widely recommended to use natural condiments and sea salt mainly.
- Saturated fats are eliminated from this plan. The intake of refined oils, like margarine, mayonnaise, etc. is restricted or limited.
- Alcohol consumption is reduced. As it has high sugar and carbohydrate content. There are some drinks that are allowed in regulated portions and in small quantities.
- The dietetic foods are eliminated preferably; since in their majority and according to several studies, they have a high content of sugar. We recommend that you read very well the labels of the products that you are

consuming, as the majority of these dietetic products are more harmful than the regular ones.

Similarly, there are many foods that can be consumed in the keto diet, most of these foods have a high content of nutrients and vitamins that restore the proper functioning of each of our organs.

As you enter this world, you will know which types of food can help you and bring certain benefits to specific organs. For example, a vegetable that is widely consumed in the keto diet is spinach. This vegetable has a high magnesium content that helps, among other things, to eliminate fatigue and it is a vital food for the brain. Just like the spinach, there are many other superfoods that, if applying this system of conscious feeding, you will get to know gradually.

Among the foods that we can consume are the following:

- The vegetables low in carbohydrates. Preferably it is recommended to consume in higher proportions green vegetables, but you can also eat onion, green onion, tomato, bell peppers, and others
- Fish. Such as salmon, tuna, sea bass, and a wide range of fish.
- Meats are also allowed either red meat, ham, bacon, chops, pork, etc..
- Eggs are widely allowed.
- Butter and creams are allowed, preferably those made with organic materials or milk from grass-fed animals are recommended.
- Cheeses are also allowed. However, the cheeses that are processed are suppressed, by which it is recommended to consume mozzarella cheese, goat cheese, blue cheese, etc...
- Healthy oils such as extra virgin olive oil and coconut oil are very commonly used as well as avocado oil.
- The condiments made naturally. Preferably it is recommended to use sea salt and Himalayan salt, also to season with green natural vegetables like green onion, and coriander, for example.
- It is advisable to consume water. In any feeding plan, the consumption of water is required for the good functioning of the intestine, and the organism in general.

- Last but not least, nuts. They must be consumed in a moderate way. The nuts that you can eat are flax seeds, almonds, walnuts, pumpkin seeds, and chia seeds.

As you have been able to observe, the ketogenic diet is strict and must be followed carefully if you want your metabolism to enter into ketosis. When this food plan is used to eliminate a disease or improve the health of a patient it is necessary to follow it strictly and rigorously so that the body can feed on energy from ketones.

Perhaps, the first few days will be complicated, but once you go through the process called keto-adaptation, you will see the wonderful benefits of practicing this diet, where you will not feel in any way the need to consume processed products, in fact, there are reports and studies that indicate that a person who reaches ketosis can fast intermittently or not with great ease because he has an inexhaustible source of energy due to the ketones produced.

The ketones as you will see in the next chapter, are an inexhaustible source of energy for the whole organism and in greater proportion for the brain. All of our organs consume a certain amount of energy, when we eat, we do not eat to provide calories to our body, but to provide energy to our organs so that each one of them can continue working correctly. And that is exactly what we want to achieve when we feed ourselves ketogenically.

Chapter 2:
What Are Ketones?

This is a concept that comes from the organic chemistry that is seen in high school. It is an organic compound, formed by a group of carbonyls attached to two carbon atoms. The first thing we are going to do is define what a carbonyl functional group is. It consists of a carbon atom that connects, so to speak, with a double bond to an oxygen atom. This type of group is obtained in soda water or blood, as you will expect. The same one is connected with two organic radicals, therefore, we can say that two free bonds are connected to the carbonyl group. These chemical connections are the ones that allow us to differentiate carboxylic acids from aldehydes, alcohols, and ethers. Ketones can be considered less reactive than aldehydes and other organic compounds.

As previously explained, ketones have a similar structure to aldehydes, since both have the carbonyl group. However, the biggest difference between them is that they contain two organic groups instead of hydrogens.

As expected, there are different types of ketones, which are divided according to:

- The structure of their chain: They can be differentiated by the structure of the chain, they can be aliphatic, because the two organic groups that are connected with their carbonyl group, have the structure of the alkyl.
- The symmetry of their radicals: This classification is used when studying the radicals, which are connected to the carbonyl group. When they are the same, as you would expect, can be called symmetrical ketones, but in the case that both are different, they are called asymmetrical, being these the most common in chemistry.
- The saturation of its radicals: Finally, another method of classification. It will depend on the saturation of its carbon chains; if they have the structure of alkenes, the ketone will be unsaturated, on the other hand, if they have the structure of alkanes, it will be called saturated ketone.

There is another type of ketone but is not characterized by any of the three previous classifications. These are called diketones because they have within their chains, two carbonyl groups in their structure. As we mentioned above, these groups are the connection of a carbon atom with an oxygen, connected by two covalent bonds.

Now, to get a little deeper into this subject, let's take a look at some properties of ketones, both chemical and physical:

Physical: Mainly, we can observe that the boiling point of these substances is much lower than alcohol's and have the same molecular weight. As for aldehydes, they do not have a big difference in their boiling point, but both have the same molecular weight.

On the other hand, ketones are soluble in water, but as the chain becomes more complex, solubility decreases.

Regarding the smell, ketones that have a small size, have a pleasant smell, medium size has a strong and unpleasant smell. Finally, the bigger ketones are odorless.

The physical state will depend on the number of carbon they possess since ketones with less than ten carbons are liquid, but those with more are solid.

Chemical: In this case, we have many more properties than in the physical ones. They are:

- Its acidity. Thanks to its carbonyl group, ketones are acid.
- Another noticeable characteristic of the ketones is their reactivity. Ketones are widely used as a product that can synthesize other compounds. For this reason, ketones can be used to make the addition of alcohol, producing hemiacetals, which are not very stable. Another addition that can be made is with ammonia and some of its derivatives, forming a group of substances called imines, which are also chemically unstable.
- They are less reactive than aldehydes.
- Ketones are difficult to oxidize and this can only be achieved with strong elements such as potassium, to say one, thus producing an acid.

Now that we have explained what a ketone is and some of its properties, we can start the book as it should be done.

As you can imagine, ketones are widely used both in industry and in everyday life. We can often find them in perfumes and paints since they are responsible for stabilizing these compounds. Sometimes they serve as preservatives because they do not allow some components of the mixture to degrade quickly. Ketones can also be used as solvents for paints and textiles, in addition to this, they are used in the pharmaceutical industry as well as in those factories that manufacture explosives.

The first thing we must ask ourselves is where to find them in nature. They are found in a lot of places such as human cortisol hormones, testosterone, progesterone, fructose, among others.

It has been proven that some ketones are found in natural sugars in really small amounts, they are found in the fructose, being it a type of sugar. The cells found on the fructose are called ketoses, which can be found on fruits and honey. Although they are ketones, the consumption of them is not recommended for the ketogenic regime, since the concentration of ketones is so small that we will not get benefit of them.

One of the functions that can be done by ketones is the biosynthesis of fatty acids; being this the purpose of the book. What is wanted with this diet is that, through ketosis, a better burning of fats is achieved. In this case, these ketones are generated due to the excessive production of the acetic enzyme. Then, the process of generating the ketone is activated, thus making the cell spread throughout the body thanks to the circulation and goes to the vital organs, such as kidney, muscles or even the brain.

But talking specifically of ketones and what they can do inside our bodies is shocking. The first thing that is done is to release the ketones when the body takes fats instead of carbohydrates as a source of energy. This manages to burn a large amount of fat. That is one of the reasons why in some diets is preferred the consumption of fat than carbohydrates. But, what does this generates?

Levels of glucose in the blood are reduced because carbohydrates become sugar for our body.

In our body, ketones have the function of burning fat to generate energy. For that reason, we recommend diets high in fats and low in carbohydrates; to force our body to generate ketones capable of generating energy. Because in the case that there is a high consumption of carbohydrates, the body will be forced to generate energy through glucose.

Since you know that ketones are cells that you need in your body, you should also guess that there should be a normal or average amount of such cells. By this, we mean that there is a level of ketones in our body which is considered "normal", as is done with other cells, such as white blood cells for example. Therefore, among the levels of ketones in the blood, are the following:

1. Less than 0.5 mmol/L: this means that there are normal levels in the blood. This level corresponds to people who have a diet that fits in normal, regarding the consumption of carbohydrates, fats, lactic, etc.. But what does this mean? Well, that the main source of energy of these people is fructose, or better said, carbohydrates, which implies that fat is not being burned, or not thanks to ketones.
2. The ketone's level in blood between 0.5 and 1.5 mmol/L: this level means small ketosis or mild ketosis. With these levels in blood, it is possible to generate energy through the process of burning fat. Nonetheless, if your goal is to lose weight, it is not yet at the appropriate level. Therefore, this level allows you to control the weight of the person.
3. The level of ketones in blood between 1.5 mmol/L and 3 mmol/L: By having this concentration of ketones in the blood we can consider that we are at the optimal level of ketosis in our body. Being this the level sought by people who make ketogenic diets. At this point, we can take advantage of the ketogenic level. Hence it is recommended to increase both physical and mental activities, in order to get the higher benefits of the keto. When this concentration of ketones is reached, our body will have a better condition to burn fat in an extremely efficient way, thus achieving weight loss.

4. The level of concentration of ketones in blood between 3 mmol/L and 8mmol/L: It is no longer good for the body since the objectives of the ketogenic diet are exceeded. At this
5. point, the results of it are not very positive because it does not have the same efficiency of using fat to generate energy. This level indicates that the body is not functioning properly. For example, the body is not sufficiently hydrated. For people who have a disease, such as type 1 diabetes, the problem may be linked to blood glucose and should be taken into account the level of insulin in their body.
6. The concentration of ketones in blood exceeds 8 mmol/L: This level is alarming since the level of concentration is extremely high for any human being. These values are not due to any ketogenic diet. These cases are found in patients with type 1 diabetes that are not controlled, being its main cause the low levels of insulin. In this case, it can be considered that the patient is in ketoacidosis due to a large amount of ketones in the blood, thus causing vomiting, nausea, and some other symptoms. This situation requires immediate medical treatment.

Already observing all the importance that ketones have in our bodies, we can say that they play a fundamental role in it. The ketones we are interested in are those generated by the liver after the decomposition of fat. But of course, this only happens at the time that the body does not have enough glucose to produce energy from it.

Chapter 3:
What Happens To Your Body When You Go Keto?

By applying the ketogenic diet as a lifestyle, our body goes into a metabolic state that is called ketosis in which our organism feeds entirely on fats.

Ketosis is nothing more than a state in which our body produces large amounts of substances, which function as a source of energy once carbohydrates are eliminated from our diet.

This could be seen as a state in which our organism guarantees its own survival without carbohydrates, learning to use fat as energy in the absence of the glucose substance. In this way our body, mainly our brain not only uses the fat stored in the blood but also feeds on the fats we eat in our food.

Differences Between Ketosis And Ketoacidosis

It is very important not to confuse the state of ketosis with the state of ketoacidosis. The second one occurs when in our organism there are excesses of ketone molecules, and the body is unable to eliminate them through urine, making our organism enter a metabolic acidity that could be considered very severe and even fatal.

Ketoacidosis could be a very frequent risk that all those who suffer from diabetes disease could suffer, being fatal for their organism if it is not treated correctly.

Benefits Of Ketosis

This condition allows our body to access fats found mainly in our bloodstream and the rest of the body. That is why it could be considered an effective way to lose weight.

Ketosis, in addition to allowing us to burn fat faster, gives us a feeling of satiety, reducing our appetite in a considerable way. In this sense, ketosis can help prevent cardiovascular disease.

- The brain: Containing high-fat substances, this provides certain curative properties for diseases such as epilepsy and even neurodegenerative diseases. Besides, has a great impact on the mood.
- In some cases, ketosis can influence diseases such as diabetes.
- Skin improvements related to the acne can be observed, as these ketone substances function as anti-inflammatory for the body.
- It can improve polycystic ovary syndrome and even fertility problems. By avoiding large intakes of insulin, the body increases androgen hormones (especially testosterone) thus increasing fertility.
- The ketogenic diet can improve glucose metabolism by lowering levels of sugar in our bloodstream and may even improve blood pressure and glycaemic profile.
- Ketonic molecules by activating our lipolytic metabolism effectively increases antioxidants in our body.
- Brain injuries: Studies reveal that this type of diet is capable of reducing some brain injuries that have been suffered as a result of an accident causing a more effective recovery in the patient. Many studies conclude that it can benefit Parkinson's and cancer patients, helping to treat some light types of these diseases and reducing the growth of cancerous tumors.

Risks Of Ketosis

Ketosis despite having its great advantages also has some side effects. That is why before starting a ketogenic diet (or any other type of diet) you should go to a specialist to examine your physical conditions and help you to develop a meal plan that can fit your needs. In this way, you will be preventing certain side effects such as:

- Sweating with a strong odor: This happens when ketone cells are eliminated.
- Bad Breath: By having excess of ketone molecules, these will be released through our breath. In the case of suffering this effect, it is recommended to consume a lot of water in order to reduce it.
- Headache: This can happen while our body adapts to our new food routine since our brain will need glycogen for its functioning. We could even feel dizziness.
- Urine with an intense odor: This happens once the ketone bodies are eliminated through the urine, which is why its odor and color can become strong.
- Lack of appetite: By decreasing carbohydrates and increasing protein and fat, our body changes the way it digests food. So we might notice that our appetite is decreasing as our body is getting used to this lifestyle.
- Arrhythmias: When so many changes take place in our organism, it is possible to show some cardiac problems.

Due to the changes that our organism suffers, it is very common that vomiting, decay, nausea, and even respiratory difficulty occur.

By reducing the consumption of fiber such as grains and cereals, we could present constipation.

Usually, this type of diet is not recommended for a period longer than three months because we could feel constantly tired and even lower our performance in everyday activities.

If we want to go back to the nutritional regime we used to have, it is important to follow the same steps we followed to start with the ketogenic diet. We must go back to carbohydrates gradually because a drastic change could cause problems such as sudden weight gain.

Chapter 4:
Heal Your Body

Everybody knows that people who make this diet seeks to lose weight. But it is also used to control some diseases. For those reasons it is important this chapter, that will talk about health.

At first, we want to give a small concept of what health is. According to the world health organization, it is "A state of complete physical, mental and social well-being, and not merely the absence of illness or injury", therefore we can say that health does not mean the absence of any disease. Instead, it means having a certain quality of life that allows us to live in a comfortable way and without so many worries. It is also contemplated to be in a good mental and social state because there are people that you may know who are physically healthy but always feel bad or are depressed. That type of person cannot be considered completely healthy, and in the long run, this has implications on their physical health.

Moreover, a small example of the implications that mental health has with physical wellness is stress because it can affect our health without us realizing. There are occasions in which we get extremely strong headaches caused by anxiety or pain. Sometimes we get muscle tension thanks to restlessness. Chest pain could be for lack of motivation or much pressure; fatigue is due many times thanks to feeling overwhelmed. Changes in sexual desire has implications with anger. Stomach discomfort can be linked to depression. Even sleep problems can be linked to all the previous problems. In addition, it has been proven that diseases such as cancer are often developed by the moods that people have, and also that the happier or mentally healthy the patient is, the better his recovery from disease is. For this reason, it is important to have good mental health, because no matter what we achieve with the ketogenic diet if we are going to have problems with our mental health.

Now that the topic of integral health is over, we can now fully focus on the benefits that keto diet has on our health.

The first thing to do is to reduce the consumption of carbohydrates, sugars and harmful fats, which affects our body for different reasons. The first two foods mentioned, become glucose and if you make a very high consumption of them; they could lead to diabetes. This does not mean that you can not consume carbohydrates, because they are one of the main responsible for energizing our body. The organs, for some of their vital functions, use the glucose into which carbohydrates are converted and thus generate many processes extremely necessary for our body. One of these processes can be when an athlete lifts weights. The muscle will need to use glucose to be able to grow or to synthesize the exercise done; but if the muscles are not able to find glucose in our body, the muscle will decrease in size, in other words, reducing body mass.

Our organs do other processes that need glucose. Nevertheless, that component can be substituted in order to do these vital functions. It is substituted by the ketones produced by the liver. An organ that satisfies these characteristics is the brain since its vital functions can be performed with ketones instead of glucose. A better example could be the previous one; muscles need glucose in order to process the exercise done. This process cannot be done by any other cell other than glucose, but if we are under the keto regime, some organ will have to donate its glucose and feed on ketones. This can be done by the brain as it is able to use ketones to perform its tasks, managing to give energy to muscles to perform their synthesis processes and not to lose muscle mass.

As you can see, glucose consumption is reduced, which means a substantial improvement in the case of people who suffers diabetes since there are some cases in which the patient can stop consuming insulin. There are also cases in which cancer patients were benefited. It is because cancer cells eat mostly glucose cells. Therefore, when eating ketogenically, the production of glucose is reduced, hence the cancer cells are unable to feed themselves. There are also some studies that reveal that the consumption of food recommended by the ketogenic diet helps patients when it comes to receiving chemotherapy or radiotherapy. Although the results are not yet conclusive, it can be said that the results obtained with the ketogenic diet are hopeful.

It is important to mention that it helps reducing overweight. Ketogenic diet's goal is to process fat and use it as energy. Therefore, when burning fat, we can lose weight, then you can lower the rates of overweight, being this one of the most common diseases in the United States and around the world.

When it comes to the brain, the keto diet is also remarkable. Thanks to the keto diet, some of the brain's functions have a better performance. First of all, it protects the brain function. According to studies, it has been discovered that the ketogenic diet could regenerate the in some occasions brain damage. These results were obtained after having done experiments on animals. The first that was done was to feed very old animals with the ketogenic diet. After some time, it could be observed that those animals who fed normally had more difficulty to perform different activities than the ones that were on the keto diet. Then, we can say that the brain works better with the ketones produced by the liver than with the glucose generated by eating carbohydrates or sugars.

At first sight, this diet can be seen as one of the bunch, which has the purpose of considerably reducing people's weight. That idea cannot be further from reality since its health benefits are incalculable. To tell one of the many benefits of keto we will go back to its beginnings. It was used in patients who suffered from epilepsy diseases; epilepsy is an electrical overactivity in some areas of the brain. There were cases in which the children did not respond correctly to the pills that were responsible for controlling the attacks. The solution was the keto diet. Amazing results were obtained as more than 10% of the children to whom this diet was prescribed stopped seizures while more than 100% of the people who suffered from epilepsy and used keto diet could reduce their seizure frequency to about half.

That was not magic, it was because this diet had very important implications related to epilepsy. When the body enters into the state of ketosis, the behavior of some genes of the brain are altered; some of them are responsible for making the energetic metabolism of the brain, thus causing seizures. Another extremely important result is that an abysmal improvement in the energy of the neurons found in the hippocampus could be observed; increasing the density of mitochondria found within the hippocampus.

As if this were not enough, it could also improve the condition of other patients who suffer from Alzheimer's, which is a degenerative disease. This disease will gradually damage the connections that occur in the brain. It affects people in a very tough way since they will lose their memory to the point of not being able to perform their daily or basic activities. But using the ketogenic diet, some of these conditions could be improved.

We cannot say that this stops or reverts the condition, but we can say that there are hopeful results when using this diet in those cases. Experimentations on animals have been made and some kind of healing and improvement were observed on their brains. Even some damage was reverted. This happens because when you enter the ketogenic state, it is possible to reactivate certain neurons and repair part of the brain damage. Additionally, we can see that it also takes care of the brain protecting the dendrites and axons improving a vital process. Dendrites and axons are in charge of brain connections so that the human body can make synapses.

Therefore, we can be sure that the ketogenic diet is not only able to make people lose weight but also allows them to upgrade their living conditions. If the patient suffers any kind of diseases such as cancer or diabetes, we can recommend to try the keto diet, obviously, with the help of an expert.

Chapter 5:
Is Keto For You?

Before trying any diet we suggest to investigate thoroughly in order to understand the consequences that it could have on our body. It is essential to know its fundamentals, advantages, and disadvantages.

It is crucial in order to know if a diet is suitable for our system or not. Because diets works differently for each person.

It is well known that this diet is low in carbohydrates, moderate in protein and high in healthy fat. That distribution is what helps us to reach ketosis; causing the liver to take fatty acids and transform them into ketones to feed itself and use them as energy sources.

This diet is based on a calorie ratio between which 60-75% covers fat intake, 15-30% covers protein intake and 5-10% covers carbohydrate intake.

Among the foods that are allowed in the ketogenic diet, we can mention fats and oils such as almonds, avocado, peanuts, olive oil, fish, pecans, and linseed. It is advisable to eat these proteins that come from an ecological origin such as meats that have been fed on grass, chickens raised in a free environment, fish and seafood, fatty dairy products such as cream, cream cheese, and cured cheeses. Among the recommended carbohydrates are almond butter, mushroom seeds, chocolate (preferably without sugar), consumption of coconut and its derivatives.

The only left step is to take into account the following aspects that could give us a preliminary evaluation to know if the ketogenic diet is convenient for our organism:

1. The keto diet has no restrictions in terms of calorie consumption, so it could be said that we could have freedom with that consumption.
2. The keto diet gives the feeling of being satisfied with meals for longer. This is very good because we do not limit ourselves to reducing our food. Instead, we feed ourselves with what is necessary and we are satisfied with it.

3. The keto diet helps us to have more energy and, although it is known that diets high in carbohydrates generate some kind of energetic decline after eating and that diets low in calories only generate hunger and stress, this diet avoids that by adapting to the fats it eliminates through the reserves and providing us with enough energy to not depend on proteins and carbohydrates. With this, we can have a high energy level during the day and we will not be constantly tired.

In few words, we can say that with the help of the keto diet we contribute to improve our physical quality of life and contribute to our health with long-term effects as long as it is done correctly. All this without worrying about the rebound effect, in which, we lose weight quickly and we gain it back in the same way. We will achieve this as long as we are willing to radically change our habits. Of course, occasionally we will be able to enjoy a pizza, a hamburger and even cookies at some meal of the day (this must be done very carefully).

The ketogenic diet is not only to feed ourselves in a healthy way, we also must be constant to get a good result. Our body will take its necessary time to process the changes and enter the state of ketosis (may occur within the first 24 hours or up to a week) and be able to begin its process of burning fat and using ketones as energy source.

If you suffer from problems tolerating certain foods high in fat, sugar problems, renal history or any other inconvenience, the ketogenic diet may adapt to your needs, but it is advisable to go to the specialist before making any change in your feeding habits.

It is important to know that ketones do not work the same way as glucose in our body and that is why we need a higher consumption of fatty acids. Doing this, the lack of glucose will be substituted, hence, fulfilling the function of reducing weight, improving our body, eliminating carbohydrates and avoiding the accumulation of useless fat.

It is well known that excess of sugars and carbohydrates are the main cause of obesity, since when fat accumulates it stagnates in our body and can cause serious problems and even have a fatal result in the long term.

All types of diet have their risks and that is why we must be attentive and know if it will fit our body because, otherwise, we can have harmful results.

It is also known that in order to enjoy good health it is important to drink plenty of water and consume varied foods in a balanced way, mostly fruits and vegetables.

Chapter 6:
Benefits Of Ketogenic Diet For Women

In both women and men, the endocrine system is formed by organs and tissues that produce hormones. These hormones are natural chemicals that, after produced, will be secreted into the bloodstream to be used by other organs. It is the general process that our endocrine system performs.

The hormones will then control those organs to which they are destined. However, there are some organic systems that contain their own systems to regulate them without needing hormones.

Now, as women (as this book is aimed for you) get older, there will be particular changes in these hormonal control systems. What is going to happen is that some organs or tissues become sensitive to the hormones that control them, in other cases, the number of hormones that the body can produce decreases with age. Sometimes, it may happen that the hormones decompose or metabolize more slowly.

Knowing roughly what happens with our endocrine system, we can deduce that when endocrine tissue ages, it can produce less amount of hormones than it was likely to, or perhaps it does produce the same amount of hormones but at a slower rate.

Among the hormones that can probably decrease over the years, is the Aldosterone hormone. This hormone is responsible for regulating the balance of liquids and electrolytes in the body. Other hormones are the growth hormone and renin hormone. In women, the levels of estrogen and prolactin generally decrease considerably over the years.

The ketogenic diet induces a metabolic condition that has been called "physiological ketosis" by Hans Krebs and has also been described as an adaptive mechanism preserved within all higher-order organisms to ensure survival during periods of starvation, illness or energy stress.

The ketogenic diet has been used with tremendous success in diseases such as epilepsy. In the case of women, most use it to lose weight and it is due to problems caused mainly by accumulated fat in the body. That accumulated fat has side effects that affect our health, so the main cause of the implementation of this diet nowadays is to lose weight.

When the processes of hyperinsulinism and hormonal alterations are occurring in women, they are not able to ovulate, considering that the entire menstrual cycle is disturbed. This is attributable to a hormonal imbalance between estrogens and progesterone; imbalance that leads to an increase in androgens which destabilizes the entire menstrual cycle and causes women not to ovulate. This increase in androgens starts to affect women's menstruation and other hormonal problems. With the keto diet, these imbalances disappear, actually, there are many gynecologists who recommend it. Surprising results have been seen in women after about ten months of following the keto diet and the evolution and improvement of the "polycystic ovary syndrome".

The entire female hormonal system improves as a result that female hormones are formed from a molecule called "cholesterol". Cholesterol is the basis for the formation of all steroid hormones like glucocorticoids, androgens, estrogens, and progesterone.

This diet is excellent for the liver and the menstrual cycle of women depends directly on hormones meaning that the keto diet helps you significantly for your entire hormonal system. As a consequence that the menstrual cycle is regulated, the ovulation improves, bleeding decreases and in fact, menstrual cramps improve significantly. In the case of women who are in menopause, the diet also helps, now that the production of female hormones is increased. Thus making this stage of the woman's life more bearable.

The keto diet improves brain health, headaches problems, and degenerative diseases. Neurologists are asking women to do the keto diet because, with the reduction of carbohydrates, migraine problems and headaches decrease and, in many cases, it eradicates the disease.

Women also notice changes in their skin such as improvements in acne by cause of reducing processed fats. Improvements have also been observed in skin color, in the decrease of blackheads, and even eye bags. That is why it is currently one of the most implemented diets in the world. All the studies that have been made, based on the diet, show satisfactory results. The life quality of each person who applies it is noticeable and that is why, when you start to apply this nutritional method, you do not want to stop it.

So to finish, we can say that, although it is quite difficult to start this diet and follow each one of the indications as it is really hard to eliminate carbohydrates and sugar from your daily foods, once your body is detoxified from all the anti-nutrients that you have consumed for many years, it will not want to return to consume these foods. When you start with these changes in your habits, your organism will enter into the state known as "keto-adaptation". After that, the changes in your body will start to occur gradually. Do not hesitate on going keto but first talk to a specialist.

Chapter 7:
Using Keto Diet To Control Or Prevent Age-Related Conditions

As the organism ages, it is exposed to different disorders. Those disorders can be both physical and mental depending on each person and their physiology. The changes that occur with age are particularly different according to each person. At the age of 20, it is very likely to have or show diseases or disorders that could be due to congenital or degenerative diseases such as multiple sclerosis, eating disorders that lead, as explained above, to cardiovascular diseases, diabetes, and some others.

From the age of 40 onwards, people tend to suffer from heart diseases and cancer, being those the main cause of deaths. Statistics especially indicate that at these ages the majority of women presents breast and pelvic cancer, and regardless of the genre, skin cancer, cancer of the colon, rectum, and prostate. From the age of 50, it is common to see cases of prostate cancer, as well as obesity, and vision problems. During their 60's, people begin to suffer from bone problems, osteoarthritis, osteoporosis, problems associated with cognitive impairment, Alzheimer's and even Parkinson's disease.

As people get old, if they do not have healthy habits, they are probably going to suffer from one of the diseases or disorders mentioned above. Sugar is an important element in these diseases, as it can alter the cellular environment of our body and thus the destruction or mutation of cells. For that reason, every day there are more and more advertisements that want to encourage citizens to opt for organic food and healthy eating, free of sugars, processed foods, and gluten.

It is difficult to think that after so many years of consuming sugar, now we have to eliminate it from our diet. But if we go back to the past we can remember that our ancestors had longer lives than the actual ones.

Visits and explorations have been made to distant towns in different countries where the entire population has life expectancies of more than a hundred years. When they were questioned about what kind of food they had, the answers were always the same. They fed with the fruits produced by nature, vegetables, tubers, meats, fish, and fruits free of pesticides, gluten, and long-lasting chemicals.

In this context, there are worldwide campaigns to raise awareness of humanity in favor of extending our lives.

The approach of the ketogenic diet goes towards those theories. The fact that we can feed ourselves with food produced by nature sounds incredible. Indeed, physiologically talking, our organism does not need carbohydrates to work, regenerate, nor to survive; neither does need alcohol nor sweets. However, they are the most consumed products these days.

The keto diet eliminates the consumption of processed sugar and this step is important. Positive changes have been observed, such as improvements in disorders coming from age, diabetes, hypertension, polycystic ovaries, Alzheimer's, Parkinson's, and other pathologies.

For this reason, although the most commonly consumed food by humans today are carbohydrates, we must lower their consumption. Their consumption produces glucose in our bloodstream and that energy is not always adequate to feed our body, as it has been observed that when the body feeds on ketones, it is better fed.

In this sense, to have a higher cellular longevity, you should feed ketogenically. This will make your body able to work with the energy produced by ketones. Up to this point, your organism will have burnt accumulated fat from our body

It should be noted that the metabolism changes at around 28 years of age. This is due to hormonal aging and progressive decrease in the production of growth hormone, and the increase in insulin.

Added to this, the food habits that are carried out at present and the lack of exercise accelerates the accumulation of fat and lowers muscle mass. This produces overweight, cellulite, flaccidity, deformities, and so on. As we can see, these hormones are fundamental in the changes produced by age, and the keto diet mainly seeks an increase in the HCG hormone and a decrease and control of insulin.

For example, one of the main problems in older adults is the loss of muscle mass. This happens as a result that the body is no longer able to generate enough glucose; for that reason, the muscles cannot use the same amount of glucose to perform the job of muscle maintenance or the increase in muscle mass when exercising. Then, gradually, due to the lack of glucose generation, the body of older people will lose muscle mass.

That is why making a diet low in carbohydrates and rich in fat, as the keto diet, will modify the way our body works. As there are processes within our body that are done exclusively with the glucose of our blood, others can be done with both ketones and glucose. Muscles use glucose exclusively, but the brain, which is the organ that consumes the most energy can use both. Therefore it consumes the most glucose in a normal food plan, but in the case of a ketogenic food plan, so many ketones are produced that it will feed on them. Because of this, the glucose stored in the bloodstream will be sent to the muscles so that they can maintain body mass.

But we have to be careful with this because we do not want to say that it is impossible to lose muscle mass since there are people who will have very positive results when maintaining muscle mass, but some will not. Saying that all people will react the same to the diet is false.

Something that happens a lot in older adults is the lack of energy. This is because, when reaching a certain age, the body does not work the same way. This can happen either because the body does not secrete the same amount of insulin anymore, so we can't burn all the glucose in our body, generating less energy; or our body does not process the food as it used, generating a lower amount of glucose in the blood that leads to a reduction of energy levels. The solution to those problems could be migrating to another meal plan, in this case, as you might expect, we recommend the ketogenic diet. To lower the consumption of carbohydrates and sugars, and to increase drastically the consumption of fats, will make you able to enter the state of ketosis, thus feeding us through the ketones that could act in a more efficient way in our body. That's why you can hear or see older adults who look very well physically since all this is thanks to food.

Statistically, there have been experiments related to longevity and the keto diet. Hopeful results were obtained, however, experiments have only been made on mice, but it has been shown that their life expectancy increases by thirteen percent due to their high-fat diet compared to those who are fed with carbohydrates. Nonetheless, the most interesting point is not only that they live longer, but they do it better since they do it free of illness and diseases.

Seeing all the benefits that can bring to older adults this type of food we can only recommend you to consume it, of course, always under the supervision of your trusted doctor It can help you to upgrade your energy and thus feel more vitalized. With this, you will have a better functioning of the brain, among other things extremely important for the proper functioning of our body.

Chapter 8:
Supporting Basic Body Systems

When we talk about ketosis, it's just a natural state that occurs when the body feeds mostly on fat when following a low-carbohydrate diet. Ketosis has benefits but also has its possible side effects.

Ketosis is the process where the body produces small energy molecules called ketones, which are known as energy for the body and are used when there is a reduced amount of sugar in blood (glucose). In the human body, specifically in the liver, ketones are produced from fats and then used as energy. The brain does not feed exclusively on glucose, therefore, we can really say that the brain burns carbohydrates when you consume them in the form of glucose, however, if you consume few carbohydrates, the brain will have no problem using ketones instead of carbohydrates. Ketosis is important because the brain consumes a large amount of energy daily, but does not feed directly from fats, it does from ketones.

This function is essential for basic survival, otherwise, as the body stores a supply of glucose product of carbohydrates from one or two days, the brain stops doing its functions after a couple of days without food. After a while, it would have to convert muscle proteins into glucose, but this process is very inefficient to maintain brain function; a situation that would cause the organs to atrophy quickly, due to the absence of food. Luckily, the human body has evolved to be more intelligent, it has fat deposits that can serve to survive several weeks, of course, this being a very extreme case. Anyways, it must be a trained person because not everyone can do it.

When the brain has the opportunity to feed on ketones made from our body fat, many people feel more energy and mental focus, which also accelerates fat burning and in turn, it tries to lose weight.

Ketosis has different benefits that it can provide to the body and the brain; one of the first benefits is to give an unlimited supply of energy, increasing mental and physical performance, and in turn, reducing hunger, facilitating weight loss without so much effort. In addition, in order for the body to enter into ketosis, it is necessary to consume few carbohydrates, effectively correcting type 2 diabetes. Ketosis has been used to control epilepsy and, even without medication, it shows great potential to treat other medical conditions such as acne, and even treat cancer.

For your body to enter into ketosis it is necessary low levels of glucose, since it is our main source of energy. That is going to force our body to look for another food, being it the stored fats in our body. To achieve this, it is essential to follow a strict diet low in carbohydrates as the ketogenic diet. To intensify the ketosis, you can effectively add intermittent fasting.

To recognize if the body is entering into ketosis, it is possible to measure it by a sample of urine, blood or breath. There are also other signs that will be seen without a test; we can say that one of the symptoms is dry mouth and increased thirst and urine.

Keto breath: this means that your body, through the breath, has a smell similar to the nail polish remover; that smell is also felt in the sweat when exercising, most of the time it is temporary. Other indicators but in a positive way, are reduced hunger and increased energy.

As has been said earlier, to achieve a state of ketosis it is necessary to restrict carbohydrates as they become glucose and the body proceeds to use it to energize the brain and other organs. But going fully into the relationship that has ketosis with the body and benefits from it, we can see the following:

- Keto diet and heart: As we all know, the keto diet is capable of making a very considerable loss of weight, resulting in burning fat in industrial quantities. That reduces cardiovascular risks as they often depend on whether the person is obese or also if he has very high blood pressure. As it lowers cholesterol also reduces the chances of having a better protection against heart diseases. Another extremely useful thing about keto diet is that autophagy is increased; it is a way of cellular cleaning, which is great to help our body. Finally, while it is true that it is required to eat few carbohydrates and many fats, it is not recommended to eat bacon every day, but with moderation. The fats that are recommended are the avocado, olive oil, and other sourced of good natural fats that are good for our body.

- Keto and the brain: In addition to the benefits we already know of the ketogenic diet and brain diseases, such as Alzheimer's or epilepsy, we can get other uses of it for the brain such as that it can increase memory capacity. It can be used in older adults or people of any age. It also helps to increase brain capacity because thanks to experiments that were conducted on fat or old animals, with the ketogenic diet they responded better than those who were not fed that way. On the other hand, the ketogenic diet has obtained positive results in people who suffer from congenital hyperinsulinism, which produces hypoglycemia; disease that could cause brain damage. At the time of using this type of feeding, many problems have disappeared in some persons. As if that wasn't enough, it has also been the solution for many patients who suffer from migraines, reducing very often the events of migraine thanks to the low-carbohydrate diet. Patients with Parkinson's have been also benefited from the consumption of the keto diet. These results were seen thanks to some studies that were conducted on this type of patients who were submitted to these diets for at least four weeks. Of those patients, forty-seven percent have reported that they feel better, and the symptoms have decreased. Finally, patients who suffered some brain damage can also visualize an improvement thanks to the ketogenic diet. That improvement attributed to the fact that it is responsible for increasing the connections between the dendrite and axons, which generates better communication between neurons, trying to regenerate the affected area.

Chapter 9:
Diabetes Prevention

Before talking about what might refer to keto in diabetes, it will be necessary to define some concepts.

What Is Diabetes?

It is known that diabetes is a disease in which the level of sugar in blood, also known as glucose, increases disproportionately. This glucose is the main source of energy in our body and comes from the food we eat in our daily meals. Insulin is the hormone produced by the pancreas to help drain that sugar in our blood and thus allow the cells to move in order to function as energy to our body. In the case of diabetic patients, the body is not able to produce insulin and in this way the glucose remains accumulated in the blood, being unable to reach the cells, causing dangerous and even deadly results for the person.

Over time, the excess of glucose in the blood can cause eye damage, damage to the nervous system, and damage to the renal system. It can also cause heart diseases, stroke and patients can even be amputated from a part of their body for damage suffered (due to excess glucose).

Types Of Diabetes

Type 1 Diabetes

This type of diabetes is one in which the body does not produce insulin on its own because of the immune system attacks and destroys the cells that are produced by the pancreas. This disease can appear at any age, but it is mostly diagnosed in children and young adults who must take a certain amount of insulin each day in order to control the sugar levels.

When a person with type 1 diabetes has a low-carbohydrate and high-fat diet, they can stabilize their blood glucose levels. However, this must be monitored constantly as it can cause hypoglycemia.

Type 1 diabetes may be seen as an autoimmune disease (the body destroys itself by mistake). You are at risk for diabetes if you have a family history of type 1 diabetes. This type of diabetes can occur at any age, but it is much more common in childhood.

Type 2 diabetes

This type of diabetes is one in which the body does not produce adequate insulin to control glucose levels. Most type 2 diabetes occurs as a result of a person who has a disordered lifestyle when it comes to food. It can appear at any age, and there are even cases of people who have been diagnosed since childhood.

A person is at risk for type 2 diabetes if he or she has had pre-diabetes or has overweight and does not do any physical activity. This disease is usually diagnosed in people over 40 years of age and in some cases, it is diagnosed in people whose family tree has had this disease.

Gestational diabetes

This type of diabetes occurs in some women during pregnancy and even disappears after childbirth in some cases. However, if a woman has had gestational diabetes, she is much more likely to have type 2 diabetes at some point in her life (either in the short or long term).

A woman is at risk for gestational diabetes if she is overweighted, older than 25, or have a family history of type 2 diabetes. It can also influence if she has the hormonal disorder of polycystic ovary syndrome.

This type of diabetes usually goes away after childbirth, but the baby is more likely to have type 2 diabetes or obesity in his or her lifetime.

As we have been talking about, the ketogenic diet is one that is based on a diet of high fat consumption, moderate protein consumption, and very low carbohydrate consumption. When our body begins to consume glucose that is stored on it, it tries to find a way to get another source of energy, which in this case would be body fat.

This is why it is considered that the ketogenic diet in addition to helping to lose weight, can help regulate glucose levels by taking advantage of excess fat found in the body. Studies have shown that the ketogenic diet can influence up to 60% in the improvement of insulin in the body.

When a person who has diabetes (regardless type 1 or type 2) avoids carbohydrates in his or her dietary routine, which are the main factor in elevating blood sugar levels, he or she may be able to decrease medications to control these levels over time. This is because by not eating food that becomes glucose, the body will be able to respond by its own to insulin.

When starting this diet it is very important to keep track of glucose levels with a specialist, because if the person takes the same dose of insulin (that was medicated before starting the diet) when eating a low-carbohydrate diet, it could cause hypoglycemia which can be very harmful to health.

As we already know, it is not possible for two people suffering from diabetes to have the same dietary approach since they may share disease, but the body's way of reacting of each one is not the same. Ketogenic diets serve the purpose of improving the digestive system by eating healthy as long as it is followed correctly. This will be connected to the patient's physical condition.

There will always be some risks that need to be taken into account if you are under medical treatment. It is very important that under these conditions the patient is fully prepared to assume a diet so demanding that should not have any fault because its consequences can be serious; causing kidney problems, hypoglycemia, ketoacidosis, and kidney diseases. It could be even fatal.

Is The Keto Diet Suitable For People With Diabetes?

Some studies have shown that the keto diet is able to improve the health of some people suffering from this disease and even, in some cases, the minority has been able to improve insulin sensitivity.

Many people see this type of diet as a therapy for the treatment or improvement of the disease; however, this result only applies to some people. Due to the different body types, different patients do not always get the same results.

A person who is not willing to follow such a specialized and strict diet is not going to be able to obtain as goods results as a person who followed this type of diet properly.

What do we mean by that?

Once explained all the factors that influence, you could conclude that the keto diet is highly recommended by experts and people who suffer from diabetes, as they have achieved very positive results in their body and other personal aspects. However, it is very delicate to follow this type of diet, because if you do not have the necessary disposition it could be very dangerous. A slight mistake can damage your health and make a lot of damage.

Can The Keto Diet Prevent Diabetes?

Some studies indicate that the keto diet might, in some way, influence the prevention of this disease (at least as far as type 2 diabetes is concerned) for the person whose purpose is to lead a healthy life. However, many times, this disease is diagnosed from childhood and any type of factor can influence (some failure in the body or possible family inheritance).

Diabetes can be prevented and (if you have it) also controlled up to a point where you will not depend entirely on medications. Of course, this will always depend on the person with the disease and their willingness to change their eating habits.

It is relevant that we are aware that when we make a type of diet in which less than 50 grams of carbohydrates are consumed per day, our body enters the state of ketosis to obtain energy through the burning of fat.

It is crucial for people with type 1 diabetes to be able to differentiate between ketosis and ketoacidosis as the last one can be dangerous because of the lack of insulin. It is also recommended to start with a low-carbohydrate diet in a less strict way (at least 50 grams per day initially) and adapt it to your taste over time.

While people with type 2 diabetes can greatly improve their health condition to such an extent that they can completely overcome the insulin injection, a person with type 1 diabetes will still need to continue injecting their insulin but maybe in a smaller amount.

Chapter 10: Dietary Exchange Through The Menstrual Cycle

All women possess hormones, which are regulated by three main glands; hypothalamus (located in the center of the brain), pituitary (located in the brain), and adrenal glands (located at the top of the kidneys). These glands are responsible for the rest of the hormones to be in proper balance, thus generating an HPA (hypothalamus pituitary adrenal axis) which is responsible for controlling stress levels, moods, emotions, digestion, the immune system, sexual desire, metabolism, and even our energy levels.

Calorie intake, stress, and physical exercise can cause these hormonal glands to become very sensitive, so it should be considered that a low-carbohydrate diet could affect the body significantly, these changes would be reflected in the attitude.

It is known that long-term stress is capable of generating very serious damage to the body, as the overproduction of cortisol and norepinephrine creates an imbalance in the body that increases the pressure on the hypothalamus and adrenal glands. This pressure causes a dysfunction of the HPA axis.

Referring to adrenal fatigue the most common symptoms that could be seen are fatigue, weakness in the immune system and a very high risk of presenting health problems.

The adrenal fatigue, being a little similar to the suprarenal fatigue has a series of symptoms, between which we can emphasize: fatigue, depressed or weak immune system, possibility of suffering hypothyroidism, inflammation, diabetes, and mood disorders in the long term; being these very serious for the health.

Many times the increase in cortisol levels is thanks to the fact that the person is submitted to a low-carbohydrate diet. As we already know, this is very different in comparison to a moderate-fat diet and for this reason, this type of diet can cause a much greater alteration of stress levels in women than in men.

By consuming few carbohydrates, in addition to generating a noticeable alteration in stress levels, could produce other discomforts such as irregular menstrual cycles or amenorrhea (this means the absence of menstrual cycle for 3 months or more). Amenorrhea is presented by the low levels of many different hormones such as the release of gonadotropin (GNRH) which is responsible for initiating the menstrual cycle and if this failed, would generate a collapse in all (or most) sex hormones, fsh, lh, estrogen, progesterone, and testosterone. Another possible cause of amenorrhea is the low levels of leptin (a hormone produced by fat cells). According to experts, it is mentioned that in women, a certain level of leptin is very necessary to maintain a normal function in the menstrual cycle in order to maintain the regular functioning of reproductive hormones.

Low calorie or carbohydrate intake may cause leptin levels to be completely eliminated, resulting in an irregular menstrual cycle. It is very common for underweight women to be the most vulnerable to low levels of these hormones. Amenorrhea usually appears after a time on a low-carbohydrate diet.

When the keto diet is made, different corporal changes are experienced; but not all of them are always negative. The keto diet could be very useful for those women who suffer from POS (polycystic ovary syndrome), this disorder is the one that suppresses the development of ovaries and the liberation of the ovules. Many of the experimental data indicate that those patients with POS who start the keto diet, manage to recover a regular menstrual cycle and can also contribute to fertility.

When suffering from POS, the excess of insulin in a woman's body is capable of causing a considerable increase in her androgen and testosterone levels, which generates a limitation in the production of estrogens and the body's capacity to ovulate.

When a woman is on the keto diet, she must prepare herself (both physically and psychologically) for the changes she is going to go through.

As mentioned above, it is quite possible that among the changes that may occur is the devastation in the menstrual cycle due to sudden weight loss (caused by alteration of the balance of estrogen and progesterone).

However, an irregular period could not be a worrying change since the menstrual cycle could stop completely; this happens a lot in women who lose a lot of weight and are very thin because their body is more vulnerable to amenorrhea (absence of menstrual cycle) due to anovulation (lack of ovulation).

It is important to note that these problems are very likely to be attributed to sudden weight loss in response to the keto diet. Otherwise, it is very likely due to other factors such as very low body mass index, a low-calorie diet and could even be presented by excess exercise; causing the decrease of some hormones that regulate ovulation, bringing consequences of irregularity.

The lack of carbohydrates could be another key factor in ovulation problems as it directly affects the luteinizing hormone which is released by the brain to help regulate ovulation. When this hormone is directly affected, hypomenorrhea (short, light menstrual cycles) may occur.

Surely you must be wondering... How many carbohydrates must a woman ingest to avoid these types of problems?

It is not really possible to indicate an exact amount since each body assimilates food intake in different ways.

In its majority, the nutritionists indicate to consume between 15 and 30% of carbohydrates, this would be the equivalent to between 75 and 140 grams daily of calories in the form of carbohydrates; nevertheless, there are cases of women in which a diet low in carbohydrates tends to benefit their organism much more (those that suffer from POS).

But, there are cases of women who are recommended to consume between 100 and 150 grams of carbohydrates a day, these can be all those:

- Mothers who are breastfeeding.
- Women who have suffered an interruption of their menstrual cycle.

- Women who wish to gain weight.
- Women who have practiced the Keto diet for a very long time.
- Pregnant women

This type of food intake will be recommended to all those women who suffer from the cases mentioned above; besides, this routine will achieve a harmony in their mood and provide a good amount of energy to perform in their daily activities.

From here, we could conclude that the keto diet can be very useful for those women who suffer from polycystic ovary syndrome which, as mentioned above, is a hormonal disorder that prevents the ovaries from releasing ovules (thus allowing a regular menstruation).

We also know that in some cases women who have made the keto diet, have managed to get a regular period, as well as helping the fertility of women.

Why is this?

This is because, with polycystic ovary syndrome, excess of insulin in the female body increases the levels of androgens and testosterone limiting the production of estrogen and also the ability to ovulate.

In conclusion, the keto diet besides promoting weight loss also helps the symptoms of polycystic ovary syndrome. It is very important to see a specialist before undergoing this diet because, as you could see it can cause a lot of hormonal changes and it is necessary to be prepared for it.

It is also highly recommended not to focus solely on the keto diet but to complement it with another style (as recommended by your specialist). So, in addition to maintaining an ideal weight, it helps you to follow this in the long term and get benefits for your body since the key to a regular menstrual cycle is to follow a diet that adapts to your needs

Chapter 11:
Ketogenic Diet And Fertility

One of the greatest illusions that women have is giving birth to a child. The great majority of women dream about it; they wish to raise him until they are grown up and want to feel proud of them. Unfortunately, not all women are capable of doing that for different reasons, as we will see below, they can be the following:

- Having untreated sexual diseases.
- Having blocked Fallopian tubes. This does not allow sperm to reach the ovule, thus not allowing the stage of gestation.
- Lack of ovulation. If the woman does not generate ovules, then it is not possible to make the union sperm-ovule, which have to unite to generate life.
- Poor quality ovules. This means that they are not able to generate a baby, no matter how many unions are made with the sperm.
- The way in which the uterus is found limits or makes it difficult to have a fertilized ovule.
- Uterine fibroids. Represents having some type of tumors, which are not cancerous, which are like walls or muscle cells, located in the walls of the uterus, they do not allow sperm to reach the ovule.
- Having an endometriosis. Meaning that you get the same tissue that covers the interior of the uterus outside it. We say this, because all the tissue that covers the inside of the uterus, also grows outside it; hence growing in places where it should not; leading to fertility problems.
- Having polycystic ovaries. This indicates that the woman has a disease, which has extremely high levels of hormones specifically androgens. This situation not only affects fertility but also affects the effect of having menstrual irregularities, acne problems and an increase in body hair.

While it is true that the ketogenic diet is not magical and it will not be able to heal all of the conditions it is true that it can help us with one of them; w with the polycystic ovaries. It is important to know perfectly the reason why it helps us and what it is about; since the explanation previously made is very ambiguous or simple. Therefore, it is better to explain it in a better way, so that we are able to talk about it properly.

The first thing is that this is a very common condition in women since it is based on a hormonal disorder in women who are at reproductive age. To start, women who have this condition have extremely irregular menstrual cycles, which can happen rarely or infrequently, or also present a period of menstruation quite long. In addition, generates an excessive level of hormone that is characteristic of men, which is called androgen. Thanks to all these conditions that can be suffered by having polycystic ovaries, small accumulations of liquid start to form. These accumulations can be blood, called follicles in the ovaries that may cause the ovules not to be generated in a normal or regular. Consequently causing fertility problems in women.

The first and very essential thing is to know if you have polycystic ovaries. This is done by observing yourself and verifying if you have a cumulus of symptoms; if you have them, it is recommended to go to a specialist doctor. Fortunately, this condition has treatment which means a great relief for women who have infertility because of the polycystic ovaries.

The first thing we can say is that these symptoms can be seen from the first menstruation happened in the woman. This occurs most of the time, but there is also the possibility that it occurs in an adult stage; nonetheless, the latter may be due to a significant weight gain. But it is important to emphasize that for you to have a real possibility of having polycystic ovarian syndrome, you must show at least two of these symptoms:

- A lot of androgen in your body. This can be seen in different ways, when we talk about the physical form, you can see to have an excess of facial hair or even body hair, but you can also see to have a lack of hair, being it a male pattern.

- Having polycystic ovaries. Which means that your ovaries are dilated, and also could have follicles around your ovules, thus causing a malfunction of the ovaries of women in an age of fertility.
- To have irregular menstrual periods. With this, we mean to present an extra menstruation that is not planned at all with the count of the twenty-eight days in order for the next menstruation to occur. It could also be a very big irregularity in the frequency that each one of your menstruations occurs; being these periods very short or very long. This can be the most common sign for the women who have the syndrome of the polycystic ovaries, this irregularity, could be that a woman has 16 or 7 menstrual periods in a year.

But the syndrome of polycystic ovaries does not appear suddenly, instead, it has some causes, this syndrome has factors which can contribute to deteriorate the situation of the ovaries as follows:

Having excess insulin in the blood: This happens, as you should know because our body is capable of processing the glucose in our body which is the main source of energy if we have a traditional diet high in carbohydrates and the hormone responsible for doing this is insulin; but as long as it is at normal levels in our body. But if this hormone is at a high level, causing the cells to be resistant to insulin, there will be a high level of sugar in the blood, which could cause an increase in androgens in our body thus producing a greater difficulty in ovulation.

Simply excess of androgen, and as we said previously, this causes a very large complication to be able to ovulate, so it becomes almost impossible to have a good fertility.

These causes can also be simply hereditary, therefore, the syndrome of polycystic ovaries can be simply because the woman has inherited this condition from her ancestors.

Little inflammation: this is measured by the production of white blood cells that generates our body, so we can combat an infection. Women who have such a condition have a type of little inflammation that will stimulate the polycystic ovaries which in the long run generate more androgens. Then, in addition to generating hormonal problems, can also generate problems generated with the heart and blood vessels.

When we see the statistics, and we observe the main causes of infertility in women, we can say that eighty percent of them have obesity, but also have insulin resistance and, as we know, having such conditions increases the amounts of androgens in our body. Being insulin resistance the major cause of polycystic ovarian syndrome. In fact, the latest statistics tell us that more than ninety percent of people who have hyperinsulinism, of course in women, have the syndrome of polycystic ovaries, being this a major problem when it comes to the fertilization process.

For this reason, we see that one of the main causes of polycystic ovarian syndrome is having high insulin, the product of having a high level of glucose in the blood and these levels of glucose in our blood are a product of a diet rich in carbohydrates or traditional food. Therefore, by making a considerable decrease in carbohydrates and sugars, we will lose a considerable amount of weight, but it decreases in a more than considerable way the level of glucose in our blood, thus decreasing one of the main causes of the syndrome of polycystic ovaries.

The first thing is that, at the time of losing weight by means of the ketogenic diet, it is possible to reduce in an extremely important way the inflammation. If you were focused enough during this chapter, you could have seen that the inflammation has a direct implication with the process of fertilization because if the woman is inflamed it is possible to get damage in the fallopian tubes, thus causing problems when fertilizing. For this reason, when making the keto diet, we can significantly lower the inflammation within our body, since this type of feeding recommends the consumption of foods that are anti-inflammatory and extremely healthy, thus achieving to lower the inflammation in our organism in such a way that we could unblock, the tube of the fallopian tubes. This will result in achieving an improvement in the possibility of getting pregnant; however, in case of having inflamed fallopian tubes, it is difficult to determine since it does not cause pain, only infertility. Therefore, a way to try to combat this condition is applying this type of diet.

On the other hand, the consumption of a ketogenic diet also allows to have better control of the hormones since the women who possess the syndrome of politic ovaries have a hormonal disorder. This disorder produces a high number of hormones that should be generated by the male gender, causing these problems in the ambit of the ovulation of the woman; for that reason, it is necessary to look for some alternatives to be able to control these hormones.

In this case, the keto diet does not stay behind and allows an exaggerated reduction in the amount of glucose in the blood which makes it possible to control insulin levels. As the person is doing a low consumption of carbohydrates, these glucose cells are not generated, thus achieving the regularization of hormones within the body of females. Moreover, there are specialists in the field that say that a decrease in weight, between five or ten percent, can involve better ovulation. With this, we can say that the ketogenic diet can help regulate hormonal behavior, leading to achieve something so wonderful like healing some women who suffered from infertility problems before doing the ketogenic treatment. There was an experiment that was made with four women, who had the illusion of being able to conceive a child but no matter how hard they tried or how many attempts they made, they had not been able. Surprisingly, after a few months of having started to eat a diet low in carbohydrates, but rich in fat, not only did they lose considerably their weight, but they also managed to rebalance their hormones, helping them to solve some of their infertility problems.

In this case, we can say that these infertility problems can be solved through the ketogenic diet, but by this, we do not mean that it can solve them all, only a few related to the syndrome of polycystic ovaries and overweight. As we have been saying through all the previous chapters, it is never too much to go to the doctor or a specialist to be able to make a treatment in which the woman is able to ovulate or to get to fertilize in order to reach the miracle of life.

Chapter 12:
Basic Recipes

As we know, the keto diet is a low-carbohydrate, high-fat diet plan. Applying this plan will make it possible to reduce weight and improve certain conditions considerably as we discussed before, like blood sugar levels and insulin levels and thus produce a transition in the body's metabolism where carbohydrates will be replaced by fat and ketones.

Now, which are the foods that we must avoid in order to successfully begin this plan?

- Cereals: corn, rice, wheat, barley, oats, grains, sprouts, amaranth, rye, among others.
- Legumes: common bean, chickpea, black bean, green pea lentil, broad bean.
- Starch: potato, carrot, yucca, sweet potato.
- Furtas: banana, papaya, apple, pineapple, orange, grape, mango, tangerine, fruit juices, nuts, fruit syrup, concentrates.
- Alcohol: beer, some wines, cocktails.
- Sugars: honey, agave nectar, maple honey, sugar, corn syrup, fructose, sugar cane.
- The foods that we should consume and that are also recommended in this diet are the following:
- Vegetables: broccoli, cauliflower, spinach, champignons, asparagus, eggplant, zucchini, brussels sprouts, lettuce, paprika, onion, tomato.
- Fats: butter or ghee, lard, homemade mayonnaise, coconut oil, olive oil, cream, dark chocolate, fatty cheeses that melt easily, avocado, nuts and seeds such as flaxseed and chia, almonds, coconut flour, coconut milk, and almond milk.
- Fruits: berries, blackberries, strawberries, blueberries, raspberries.

- Proteins: tuna, ham, chicken, turkey, eggs, sausage, salami, beef, pork, veal, bacon, fish preferably oily fish, duck, and seafood.
- Canned food can be consumed but you will first have to carefully read the ingredients and verify that they do not contain sugars, corn syrup or starch.

Once we have knowledge of the foods we should not eat and those that we should consume we can proceed to know some of the basic keto recipes. In this order of ideas, we are going to proceed to show some short but delicious simple recipes that we can prepare to begin to change our life plan and our diet.

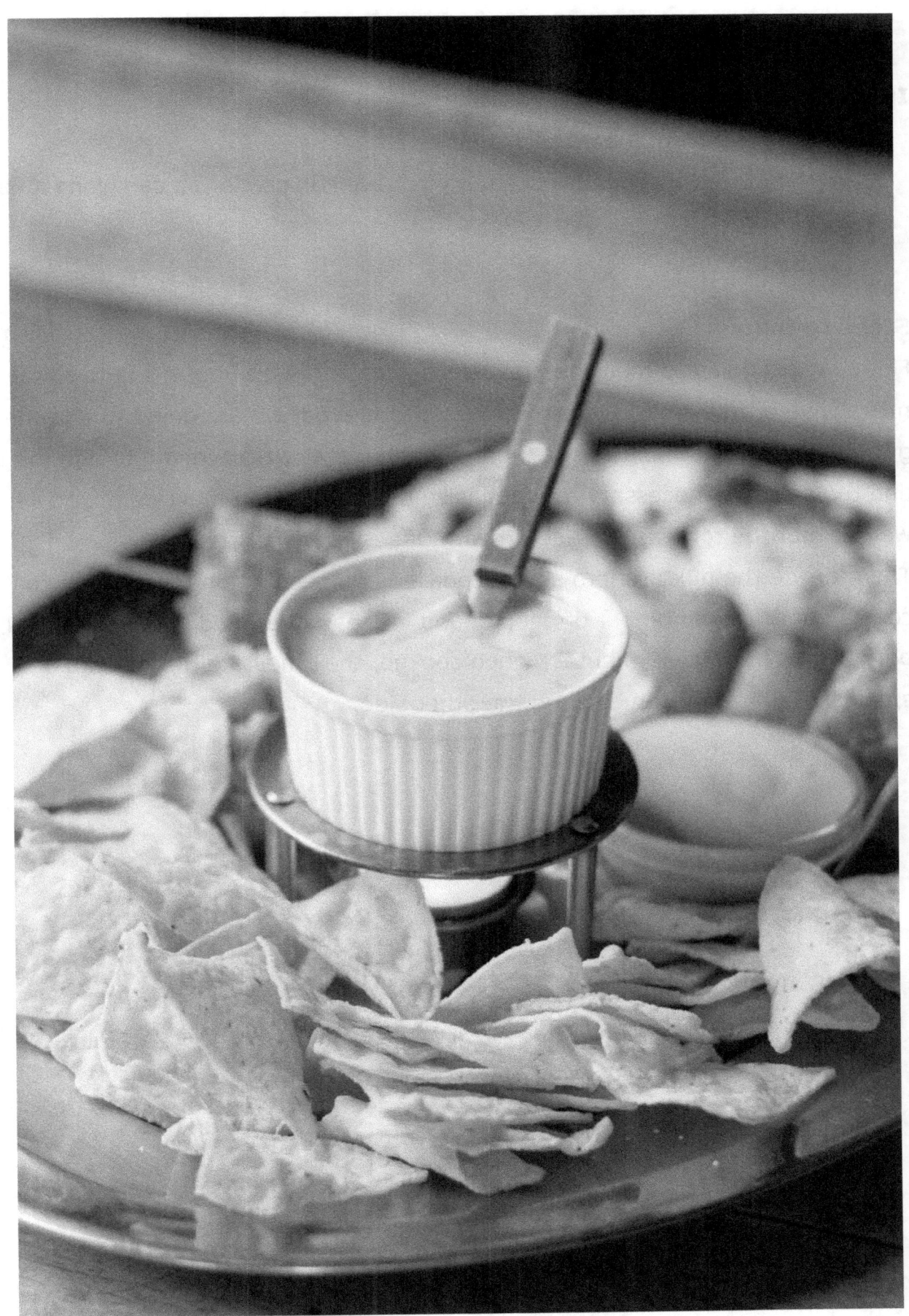

Keto Tortillas With Linseed

Ingredients:

- 300 grams of mozzarella cheese.
- 50 grams of ground linseed, if you have it in seeds you can blend it easily.
- 1 egg.
- Salt to taste.

Steps to follow:

First, we are going to melt the mozzarella cheese (we can do this in the microwave or in a satin). Once the cheese is melted, we are going to add the ground linseed and mix the two ingredients. Finally, we are going to add the egg and the salt. It is necessary to emphasize that everything must be mixed very well so that the tortillas are not left with undesired consistences.

Then, divide the mixture into several portions, depending on the amount that comes out and the number of people, and in a pan over medium heat extend the portions for about five minutes; when cooked, they must be turned with a spatula so that they can cook on the other side.

Keto Tortilla With Almond Flour And Coconut

Ingredients:

- ¾ Cup of almond flour.
- 4 spoonfuls of coconut flour.
- 1 egg.
- Salt to taste.
- 2 spoonfuls of warm water.

Steps to follow:

Place all the ingredients in a bowl, mix and knead until you get a homogeneous dough that is wet to the touch because we do not want it to be liquid to be able to manipulate it.

If we see that the dough is too dry, we can add a little water and knead again and this way you will work with the consistence you want to.

Once you have the dough with the desired consistency, wrap it in a food plastic and let it rest for about 10 minutes.

Once it has rested enough time, we proceed to divide the dough in about eight portions or in the quantity that is wanted, according to the size of the tortillas that are wanted to make.

The tortillas can be given the round shape either with palms with the hands in a natural way or can be made with the tortilla machine or with a bakery roller, if available.

If we make it with the method of the palms, we are going to place the balls of dough in a waxed paper and it will be given the round form with the palms of the hand.

With the machine for tortillas, you will place the ball of dough in the middle with the waxed paper so that it does not stick and crush until you get the tortilla.

Another way is to place the dough balls in the middle of two sheets of wax paper and stretch them with the roller until they acquire the shape, size, and thickness we want.

If we want them to be totally round we can make use of the cutters that are used in pastry.

Later we will proceed to place them in the frying pan (preferably anti-adherent) to medium heat, and let cook for 30 seconds approximately or when we observe that it begins to cook and change color. Then, we turn them to cook on the other side for a few more seconds and so on until you finish the desired amount of tortillas.

EMPANADAS OF KETO MEAT

Ingredients:

For the dough:
- 1 ½ cup almond flour.
- 1 ½ Cup of mozzarella cheese.
- 100 grams of cream cheese.
- 1 egg.

For the Stuffing:
- 1 tablespoon of butter preferably Ghee or clarified.
- ½ Kg of ground beef, you can perfectly mix it with a little pork meat and it will give it a surprising taste.
- 1 tablespoon finely chopped onion.
- ½ chopped tomato.
- Salt to taste.
- Ground pepper to taste.
- Concentrated consommé of beef broth, this is optional to add some more flavor.

Steps to follow:

1. In a frying pan over medium heat add the butter, you can add a little chili if desired, onion, tomato, and let's fry for a few minutes over medium heat until you see that your ingredients are integrating and cooking.
2. Then add the meat, mix, season with salt and pepper to taste, and if we have beef broth, we add it and let all the ingredients cook and mix for about five minutes approximately or until you see that the ingredients are well mixed and cooked.
3. We are going to let the meat cook a little and dry, but not much so that it is a little juicy, then we are going to let it rest to use it to fill the dough and make empanadas.

For the dough:
1. Mix the cream cheese and mozzarella cheese in a bowl, we can melt the cheeses in the microwave or manually in a pot, the important thing is to melt them so they can mix well. After we have mixed the cheeses, we add the egg, mix well to add almond flour gradually, and we are going to mix until a manageable dough is obtained, then let it rest for a few minutes.
2. To make the empanadas we make a few balls, the size will depend on the size we want our empanada. Again, we can make tortillas with the palm of the hands, with the machine to make the tortillas or in its defect with the roller, as explained in the previous recipe.
3. Once the tortilla has been made, add the meat filling that we left to rest earlier. Fold the tortilla in half and seal the dough with the fork so that the filling does not come out.
4. Then place the empanadas in a tray with waxed paper and take it to the oven at 180 Celsius degrees for 15 minutes or until they are golden. And they are ready to taste.

Keto Pizza

Ingredients:

- 200 grams of almond flour.
- 700 grams of grated mozzarella cheese.
- 75 grams of cream cheese.
- 2 eggs.
- 150 grams of salami.
- 150 grams of Pepperoni.
- 150 grams of ground beef.
- 50 grams of Ghee butter.
- 50 ml of unsweetened tomato paste.
- Salt to taste.
- Ground Oregano to taste.
- Garlic powder to taste.

Steps to follow:

1. The first thing we are going to do is preheat the oven to 200 Celsius degrees while we prepare the dough and pizza.
2. For the dough, we are going to melt the cream cheese and half of the mozzarella cheese, we can melt it as it is already known in the microwave or in a pot avoiding of course that the cheese burns. It only has to reach the necessary temperature so that it melts and the two cheeses can be mixed.
3. Once the cheeses are mixed we add the salt to taste, the almond flour, the eggs and we mix everything very well, only in case it is necessary to be able to achieve a better mixture we can place again our container in the microwave to melt the cheeses and to mix well.
4. In a pizza mold, place a waxed paper to prevent our dough to stick; we are going to extend the dough in the pizza mold. A way to extend perfectly the dough is with this technique: we are going to place the dough in the waxed paper and on top, we are going to place another sheet of waxed paper and stretch. Once reached the desired size remove the waxed paper from above and take the mixture to the oven for about 10 to 15 minutes at a temperature of 200 ºC until we see that it begins to roast a little.

5. For the filling of our pizza, we are going to stir fry the meat with the butter or if we prefer we can do it with olive oil.
6. Once the base of the pizza is golden brown, remove it from the oven and let it rest so that the cheese solidifies, then add the tomato paste mixed with garlic powder and oregano, add the ground beef, pepperoni, sliced salami, and finally the rest of the mozzarella cheese.
7. We put it back into the oven; this time for a few minutes because all we want is to melt the mozzarella cheese, let cool a little and it will be ready to eat. If we want, we can also add olives and mushrooms.

Keto Cream Of Mushrooms With Spinach

Ingredients:
- 1 clove of garlic.
- ½ Medium onion.
- 250 grams of natural preference sliced mushrooms.
- 1 tablespoon Ghee butter.
- 300 ml of whipping cream.
- 1 cup spinach.
- 1 pinch of salt to taste.

Steps to follow:
1. In a frying pan over medium heat add the butter and cook the finely chopped onion and garlic. When the onion has a transparent color, add the sliced mushrooms and stir constantly so that they do not stick until they are golden and caramelized.
2. Then we will add the whipping cream, the pinch of salt, and move carefully to incorporate until it boils.
3. When the boil breaks, add the spinach, stir and let cook for about two minutes so that the spinach is not overcooked.

4. All we have to do now if we want to; is to blend all the ingredients to obtain the cream. There are people who do not blend it and the flavor is just as wonderful, once the cream is obtained we serve it hot and enjoy.

5. If we get leftover cream, we can refrigerate it in a container with lid and save until the next time we want to consume, at that time, it can be heated in a frying pan over low heat. This recipe can also be used as a sauce to complement a chicken or pork and is equally delicious.

As we can see, it is easy to take this food plan and once we try the recipes we will realize that they are as tasty as the usual diets. It is crucial to try that the food is accompanied by nutrients that our body can absorb, such as spinach and vegetables, coconut oil and other foods that provide a good amount of vitamins and nutrients necessary for our body.

Chapter 13:
Food Choice

It is already known to us that if we eat the right diet we can reach the desired levels of ketosis and enjoy the many benefits that this provides.

That is why it is important to evaluate very well which foods we are going to buy when starting the ketogenic diet. The important thing is to choose products that, in addition to being allowed in the keto diet, provide us with the vitamins and minerals that our body needs because, as the cellular environment is regenerated and cleaned, we will have the ability to absorb all the nutrients from the food ingested.

Based on this, we are going to talk about some foods that are supposed to be consumed in this diet for the nutritional contribution they have for our body.

Whitefish, such as hake or similar fish are a good choice as they are lean options and very reduced in calories but with a high-quality protein for our body, especially for its high proportion of omega 3, essential for health.

The avocado is one of the few oily fruits sources of vegetable protein admitted by the keto diet and also widely used in this food plan for its big versatility when preparing a dish as it is used for salads, sauces, and even desserts. The avocado is a fruit considered an excellent antioxidant and rich in vitamins and minerals, with a natural fat that is widely used in these keto diets.

Vegetables are also allowed and widely recommended in the ketogenic diet; especially green vegetables. These green vegetables are source of vitamins and recommended fibers; in the specific case of spinach we have that it is a vegetable used in most keto dishes and it is because spinach, apart from containing fiber, has vitamin A, B1, B2, C, K, calcium, phosphorus, iron, folic acid, is rich in magnesium, zinc, and beta-carotene, the latter slowing the action of free radicals, making spinach to be considered as a natural anticarcinogen. Spinach can improve the functioning of the immune system and vision. As we already know, vegetables form most of the distribution of food that must be present in the daily dishes so it is necessary to ingest products of good quality and with a great contribution such as spinach.

In the case of vegetables, not all vegetables are allowed in the keto diet, this is because some of them have a high content of starch and carbohydrates that are processed by the body as sugar and, as far as we know, we must avoid it in this diet plan. That is the case of the potatoes, sweet potatoes and cassava, for example. However, there are other vegetables that are allowed since they are low in carbohydrates, such as cauliflower, broccoli, bell pepper, celery, cucumber, eggplant, and asparagus. Cauliflower is a highly recommended and used vegetable, low in carbohydrate and high in fiber and vitamin C.

When talking about cheeses, the first thing we are going to recommend is to consume organic and defatted cheeses coming from animals preferably fed with grass. It is important to be able to evaluate the nutritional information of the cheeses that are ingested, the lesser ingredients they have the better they are since there are many products that can have stabilizers that add carbohydrates and sugars to the cheeses.

A topic of discussion is the consumption of milk as it contains large amounts of carbohydrate so the milk allowed is from nuts; such as almond milk, and coconut milk without sugar. The detail is that many specialists do not recommend consuming those milks because to generate a glass of almond milk, it requires large amounts of almonds, thus exceeding the amount of fat you can ingest daily. You consume large amounts, of course, that is what it is recommended in the keto diet, but moderately. The same applies to almond and coconut flours. In the case of clarified butter or Ghee, just like the oils allowed, its content is clearly fat without carbohydrates or proteins. In fact, more than 60% of the ketogenic diet is fat, so they are one of those that can be used with more confidence for the preparation of most dishes. It is recommended, as we have been saying previously, to choose good quality products and, currently, on the market there is a wide variety of them.

Nutritional yeast is a good ally of people who apply the ketogenic diet because when it is sprinkled on meals you get a delicious cheese flavor, it is also rich in vitamin B12 and is often used to make cakes and breads.

Another component of food that we can not leave behind and that we want to recommend is collagen. This can be found in the gelatine extracted from the broth of beef legs, for example. Collagen is the most abundant protein in mammals including humans. It is one of the most important components, especially in these processes in which people are losing weight and reducing sizes and is required to improve the elasticity of the skin. Collagen helps the skin, bones and connective tissues and represents almost a third of our total mass of protein.

That is why we strongly recommend consuming gelatine that is collagen in a natural way. The most commonly used is the gelatine made with beef legs broth, which contains a large amount of collagen protein.

There is an oil used in the ketogenic diet that has many properties and it is the MCT oil, it consists of concentrated caprylic acid and which is 8 times more concentrated than coconut oil.

MCTs are easy to absorb fatty acids that metabolize very quickly and are effectively converted into long-lasting energy for the brain and body, and help to increase energy, endurance, and mental concentration while in a low-carbohydrate or ketogenic state.

MCT oil increases metabolism and improves your body's ability to burn body fat as a fuel source. As MCT oil is naturally tasteless and odorless it can be easily mixed with food without altering its flavors. For those who are starting to consume this type of oil, it is advisable to start with half a teaspoon that can be added to the morning coffee or in the coffee with which you are going to break the fast for example.

The Himalayan Pink Salt is another good recommendation that you can add to the amount of products that you must acquire if you are going to start this diet since it is a salt that preserves all the essential minerals and electrolytes, promotes healthy pH levels in the body, contains natural iodine, improves circulation, and does not increase blood pressure. Otherwise, common salt is not recommended because its minerals are lost in the process of industrialization and it can cause high pressure in the body when consumed in excess; iodine in this type of salt is artificially added in and it also includes anti-glomerate compounds. So when consuming salt in our meals choose pink salt or Himalayan salt.

With all that we have been able to appreciate so far, we have that within the great variety of foods allowed, if we evaluate and investigate their enormous properties and, in addition, we look for different combinations of dishes or menus that we can do with them, we will not find ourselves in the need to get bored of this lifestyle. We have to learn why some vegetables, for example, are not allowed in the food plan, only in this way and acquiring the knowledge about nutritional content of each of the foods we consume, we acquire awareness and responsibility of not consuming it.

Let's talk about cereals. They have a certain quantity of starch, some have more than others, that are metabolized in our body in the form of sugar; something that we should not consume in the keto diet. So, this type of food should be avoided, such as the case of rice, and we can replace it with keto rice using cauliflower. There is a wide variety of options that we can do and try to adjust the plan, not only to our economic needs but also to the needs and requirements of our body.

In the case of alcohol, it is not recommended to consume beer, cocktails and some wines. In the ketogenic diet, some types of wines may be allowed, such as dry wine containing less than 0.5 grams of sugar per glass. Most wines are presentations of beverages with carbohydrate concentrations due to various fermentation processes such as glycerol, which has a minimal effect on blood sugar concentration or insulin levels. With this information, we can use the analogy that every time we consume a glass of wine we are drinking 2 grams of carbohydrates.

When applying the keto diet, if we want to achieve the benefits and be able to obtain the levels of ketosis; we must not only be aware that we must follow the indications of the ketogenic diet, but also have some examples and some knowledge that we must take into account when choosing foods. Knowledge like: which vegetables are not allowed and which are the consequences of their consumption. We must also evaluate which foods we will consume and why, what benefits it would be contributing to my diet. If we do this process in a planned way organizing a weekly menu, for example, we can achieve our goals easily.

As it has been reiterated on several occasions, this type of food should be monitored by a nutritionist or expert in the area because each body reacts differently and the requirements of one person are not the ones of another person. In addition, each person may have different inflammatory problems or food allergy that should be considered before starting any diet. Although the keto diet is wonderful and has a wide variety of proven benefits, it is also true that each person should be evaluated by an expert.

Chapter 14:
Breakfast

When practicing a traditional eating plan (with this we mean one that has a normal intake of carbohydrates) it is said that breakfast is one of the most important meals of the day as people go a long period without eating food from the night of the last day. This implies that this is the first meal of the day; the one that allows people to get enough energy to face their day with all the challenges it can have. If you do not eat breakfast, and then eat lunch, for example, it is very likely that people will feel hungry throughout the day.
For the reasons stated above, it is important to show you some recipes in order to have a good ketogenic breakfast.

Cups Of Egg, Ham, And Cheese

This is a very simple recipe, as you do not need many ingredients. They are cheese, ham, and eggs; these are ingredients that can be found in every fridge. Besides, this is not very complicated to prepare since you do not have to be a chef to make it. In addition, it can also be done very quickly, in an approximate time of twenty-five minutes. So, if you are in a hurry for the daily struggle, this recipe is very good for you. The ingredients are as follows:

- A spoonful of butter.
- Twelve slices of ham.
- A cup of shredded cheddar cheese, or a cheese that is fatty.
- Twelve large eggs.
- Salt to taste.
- Pepper to taste.
- Freshly chopped parsley.

When we see these ingredients, we can see that the recipe does not require anything out of the ordinary. Hence, anyone can make this recipe and as you will see below, it is not a very difficult process.

1. Preheat the oven at 400°.
2. Grease a tray of muffins with butter; you are going to grease the cavities of the muffins.
3. Place the slices of ham inside the muffin cavities covering them with the ham.
4. Place the cheese inside each cavity, above the ham that has already been placed.
5. Break one egg per muffin cavity on top of the cheese.
6. Season with pepper and salt to taste.
7. Decorate with parsley.

By observing how it is prepared, you can see that its preparation is extremely simple, for that reason, you can cook it without the need for having advanced knowledge in the kitchen. All you have to do is to preheat an oven, and then put ham, cheese, and egg; then wait until everything is ready. This recipe is very simple, but at the same time, it is very tasty.

Stuffed Peppers

For this recipe, not much is needed, only bell peppers and eggs. Obviously, you can add the ingredients you want, as long as what you want to add is allowed in the ketogenic diet. This recipe is as simple as the last one, but in this case, instead of using molds for muffins, we will be using the bell peppers.

The ingredients are as follows:
- Two large bell peppers, halved and seeded.
- Eight beaten eggs.
- A quarter of a cup of milk.
- Four strips of bacon, cooked and toasted, cut into small squares.
- One cup shredded cheddar cheese.
- Two tablespoons of scallions, finely chopped.
- Salt to taste.
- Pepper to taste.

As you could see, the recipe doesn't need many ingredients, and the ones you need are very common, therefore, for you to make this breakfast, you don't need many things. If that wasn't enough, the process to cook this breakfast is extremely simple.

1. Preheat the oven at 400°.
2. Place the peppers on a baking tray facing up and add a little water.
3. Put the peppers in the oven for about five minutes.
4. Beat the eggs and milk until smooth.
5. Add bacon pieces, cheese, spring onion, salt and pepper to taste.

6. Pour the mixture into the peppers, and leave them in the oven. Leave about thirty to forty minutes in the oven.

As you can see, this recipe is extremely simple and does not need much more than simple ingredients. This recipe consumes a little more time than the other one, but it is worth it, so we can only recommend you to cook it and try it.

Chapter 15:
Lunch

Lunch is a vital meal for the human being, even despite being in a ketogenic diet, it is always important to eat three meals a day. Skipping one of the three main meals affects the metabolism of each person.

To be able to make such a diet, and not suffering in the attempt, we will recommend you to make the following recipes:

Cobb Egg Salad

Eating salad is always good, for that reason, we recommend you to eat it. It has different foods rich in fats; they are foods such as bacon or avocado that has natural fats which help our body to enter ketosis. The ingredients are as follows.

Ingredients:

- Three tablespoons of mayonnaise, preferably natural.
- Three spoonfuls of Greek yogurt, since it is the healthiest of all.
- Two spoonfuls of red wine.
- Kosher salt.
- Black pepper to taste, as this doesn't affect the ketosis process.

- Eight boiled eggs, you can chop as you wish, it is recommended to chop them into several round pieces for decoration, but if you are a person who does not care about the appearance, chop them as you like. That amount is the minimum, but you can use the amount of boiled eggs you want.
- Eight strips of bacon, which you can cut into strips or squares. At the time of cooking, this amount is recommended as a minimum, but you could consume more bacon, so you can decorate the Cobb egg salad.
- An avocado that should be cut into thin strips. You can cut it as you like either as squares or strips and you can consume the amount of avocado you wish.
- Half a cup of blue cheese shredded or crumbled, this the cheese is not exclusive, you can consume the cheese you want, such as smoked or yellow cheese as long as it is high in fat.
- Half a cup of cherry tomatoes, the same chopped in half. If you do not have this type of tomatoes, you can also eat regular tomatoes, chopped in small squares.
- A quantity of two tablespoons of chives chopped very small.

Now, the preparation process is very simple, only two simple steps are needed.

1. In a small bowl add the mayonnaise, the Greek yogurt, and the red wine, stir well until you have a homogeneous mixture, after having done that, proceed to add salt and pepper. This step is responsible for making the sauce, or rather the salad dressing.
2. Then, in a larger bowl, we proceed to add the eggs, bacon, cheese of your choice and cherry tomatoes; after they are all there we proceed to gradually add the dressing previously made, it is going to be added until all the ingredients are well covered with it, after that, try the salad and proceed to add salt and pepper to taste. Finally, add the chives to decorate the salad to taste.

As you could see, the process and the ingredients to make this salad were really very simple. The preparation should not take more than ten minutes since you only need to chop the vegetables, cook the bacon, make the eggs, and mix well, which should not take much time nor knowledge in the culinary field.

Stuffed Avocados

This is a very simple and fast recipe, for which you do not need many ingredients. All you need are avocados, onions, fatty cheeses, nothing too exotic or very difficult to get because you only need things that you can get in your home market. Besides, you do not need to be a chef since this recipe is extremely simple; on the other hand, if you are in a hurry you won't waste a lot of time either since the time it will take you to prepare this recipe is between ten minutes or a little more. The recipe quantities are equivalent to about four portions for people who do not eat a lot, but for people who are used to eat a lot, could serve as two portions.

The ingredients are the following:
- Four avocados that are well ripe.
- The juice you can get from a lemon.
- A spoonful of olive oil, preferably extra virgin.
- An onion of medium size, which is chopped as you prefer.
- One pound of ground beef.
- Condiments of your preference to prepare the tacos. Moreover, there are packages made for you to prepare the tacos.
- Kosher salt to your liking.
- Black pepper, fresh and freshly ground.
- A cup of yellow cheese, or also Mexican shredded cheese.
- Half a cup of chopped lettuce.
- Small chopped cherry tomatoes, or regular tomatoes chopped in small squares.
- Sour cream, for consistency and decoration.

After having all these ingredients, we can proceed to the preparation but it should be noted that to make this recipe; the ingredients we just mentioned are the basic ones so if you want to add more ingredients you can do so. As long as you do not go out of what stipulates the ketogenic diet, which is not to consume carbohydrates or sugars. Well, explained that point, we will proceed to explain how to make its preparation.

1. We take our avocados and chop them in half, we take out the seed, boning the avocado, thus leaving as a hole in the avocado, which is the space occupied by the seed. Finally, we put lemon juice to our avocados, to prevent them from oxidizing.
2. Then, place in a frying pan over medium heat the oil until it is bubbly, at that time, that the oil is very hot, add the onions that had already been chopped. Let them cook until they are golden, this may take a little bit, about three or five minutes.
3. Add the ground beef and the seasoning of your preference; then, with the help of a wooden spoon, move the meat, also keep seasoning with salt and pepper. Afterward, the beef is going to be put together in the pan with the onions. Cook until the meat is not pink, this meat cooking lasts about five or six minutes.
4. After the meat is cooked, drain the fat from it.
5. After draining the meat, proceed to grab the avocado and fill in the avocado holes with all seasoned ground beef. Finally, at the top of the stuffed avocado, add the cheese, tomato, lettuce, sour cream and enjoy your meal.

As you could see, in order to make the avocado tacos recipe you don't need to be a chef. It only takes a little time, and it's not much since it should take about ten minutes, therefore, this recipe is extremely effective when you are busy or in a hurry. Besides, it will allow you to continue with a keto lifestyle without losing or skipping good meals because practicing this style of food, does not mean eating badly or insipid, it is quite the opposite.

Keto Bacon Sushi

For lovers of Asian food, especially those of sushi, we have this dish, which is not really sushi but it has its form because when preparing it, we will give it the shape of them. It is very similar to the traditional sushi, but a ketogenic one. No special ingredients are needed either, because you can use carrots, bell peppers, among others. It is also important to say that this recipe will also provide a perfect balance, as you will eat vegetables and some fats. The estimated time to make this recipe, adding the time to chop all the ingredients, and then cook them, is half an hour, therefore, although we could see an increase in time when cooking the recipe, we can also see that we are expanding our menu with simple recipes.

The ingredients are as follows:
- Six slices of bacon, the same chopped in half, to then be able to use them to make the covering of the pieces of sushi. The bacon in this recipe will act as the seaweed, which will cover the sushi.
- Two cucumbers, it is recommended that the same are chopped into thin slices.
- Two medium carrots, it is also recommended that the carrots are chopped into very thin slices.
- Four ounces of cream cheese, quite soft, so that after it can be mixed with other things.
- Sesame seeds to decorate.

After having the ingredients chopped and everything ready, we proceed to begin the cooking process, but not before specifying that we can make keto sushi with any vegetable, in this case, we are using carrots, but they can be replaced by bell peppers to say something different than carrots. Now, let's get to work.

1. The first step is to preheat the oven to four hundred Celsius degrees.
2. We take some of our trays, which we use for baking and we will wrap it in aluminum foil.

3. Place the bacon on top of the aluminum that has covered your tray, so that it can be cooked. It must be placed in such a way that the halves of the bacon are in a symmetrical way or better said, place the bacon so as to create a uniform layer. They should be baked until the bacon is crispy but also that a little easy to fold, possessing a certain grade of flexibility.
4. Then cut the carrots, avocados, and cucumbers to the same width as the bacon.
5. After the bacon has rested so that you can touch them with your hands, you will proceed to put a little cream cheese on top of the ends of the bacon and proceed to take the vegetables that you had already chopped and place them evenly on it. Preferably, place those vegetables at the ends of the bacon.
6. Roll up the vegetables quickly and tightly with the bacon.
7. Finally, we proceeded to decorate the recipe with seeds of alamo to the taste of each guest.

As we could see with this recipe, which sounds delicious, you don't need a lot to eat delicious, you just need imagination and a little time. As we said previously, vegetables can be replaced, not only we can make keto sushi with carrots, we can also use tomatoes, bell peppers, cucumbers, among other foods. You just need imagination to make this recipe more diverse and more delicious.

As you could see in this chapter, with these three recipes of ketogenic lunches, you will not lose the quality of your food, only that you will not consume carbohydrates. With this, we mean that your food will not lose flavor. Instead, it will maintain it, therefore, you will not find it difficult to migrate to this type of ketogenic food since as you can imagine, the flavor is delicious and you will be feeding better, cellularly speaking. What we can tell you is to try these recipes, investigate new and different recipes to make variated lunches, and create your own ones.

Chapter 16:
Dinners

Generally, dinner is a dish that is difficult to plan. Perhaps we spend all day in most cases in the street and when we get home we do not want very elaborated or difficult menus. Nevertheless, there will be special occasions in which we will have time to prepare a delicious dinner. For those who practice fasting, probably this is their second meal of the day, for those who don't, we talk about the third meal of the day. Regardless of the case, we must take into account that at the evening meal it is recommended not to consume or reduce to the maximum the consumption of carbohydrates. In this order of ideas, we will give some recipes for dinner following the ketogenic style.

Breasts Stuffed With Pesto Sauce And Mozzarella Cheese

Ingredients:

- 3 breasts
- 250 grams of Mozzarella cheese approximately, if you like a lot of cheese add more.
- A large fresh bunch of basil.
- 1 clove of garlic
- Olive oil to taste
- A handful of almonds
- Shredded Parmesan cheese to taste.
- Salt and pepper to taste

Steps to Follow:

1. Wash the basil leaves well and add them to the glass of the blender. Now add the almonds and the whole peeled clove of garlic. Then add 3 to 4 tablespoons of olive oil, a little salt, and pepper to taste and proceed to blend. We must obtain a creamy emulsion; if we see that it lacks more liquid, we can add more oil until it reaches the point that more pleases us to the palate.
2. We must ensure that everything (especially the garlic) is well crushed.
3. When the sauce is ready, blended, and with the desired consistency, add the Parmesan cheese and, if you want, blend again at medium speed, there are people who do not blend the cheese and can do so as well.
4. Now with this delicious pesto, we are going to fill the breasts.
5. We are going to open the breasts like books, and we are going to add salt and pepper to taste.
6. We add a good and appetizing layer of the pesto we already prepared and later we place several slices of Mozzarella cheese on top.
7. Roll up the breasts and hold them with sticks of wood or bamboo.
8. We can cook them in the oven or in a non-stick frying pan. And the tasty dinner of breasts stuffed with pesto and Parmesan cheese is ready.

Hake With Romesco Sauce And Vegetables

This dish is ideal for the night when you want to make a more elaborate meal. The sauce is ideal to accompany both fish and chicken as the case may be. This recipe is designed to get a thick sauce, you can make it more liquid if you like. Here I use the hake but you can choose the fish you want.

Ingredients:
- 1 ¼ Cup of Almonds
- 2 cloves garlic
- 500 grams of bell peppers
- 3 Tomatoes
- 1 Gren onion
- Half Onion or a medium Onion.
- Olive Oil
- Salt to taste
- Pepper to taste
- 3 Hake

Steps to follow:
1. First, let's make the sauce. Cut the bell peppers into pieces and process them together with the tomato, onion, garlic, and almonds; you have to process them very. We are going to process for about 30 seconds; when we are processing everything we add about three or four tablespoons of olive oil. We see the consistency as we process the mixture. When we say process we mean to cook.
2. When the sauce is ready we proceed to make the hake, once cleaned and filleted we add a little lemon, this step is optional according to the taste of each one, but the seasoning with lemon gives a wonderful aroma and flavor to the fish. Then we are going to season with salt and pepper. And we are going to place them in a frying pan, preferably non-stick, and cook

carefully over medium heat until they are ready. Obviously, we will have to turn them so that they cook on both sides.

3. Once ready and served, add the romesco sauce on top of the hake.

If you wish, you can accompany it with avocado and stir-fried bacon, it is a wonderful combination for this dish.

Broccoli And Sausage Tortilla

It is a simple dish to make for dinner and within the standards of the ketogenic diet. If you like it you can add more vegetables to it.

Ingredients:
- 1 large whole broccoli.
- 2 or 3 sausages; should be organic chicken, preferably pre-cooked.
- Clarified Butter or Ghee.
- 6 large eggs preferably.
- Fresh oregano, chopped parsley.
- Salt to taste.
- Pepper to taste.
- 1 avocado.

Steps to follow.

1. The first thing we are going to do is to cook the broccoli. It is recommended to boil the water first in a pot and once the water is boiling we are going to place the broccoli in a period of about 3 to 5 minutes since we do not want it to be overcooked. Actually, it will be better al dente. Once cooked the broccoli, we submerge it in ice water to stop the cooking, and later we chop it in small pieces and add salt to taste.

2. In a frying pan add ghee butter and the sausages that were previously thinly sliced and cook them. When they are ready, add the broccoli, fry it together with the sausages and add salt, oregano, finely chopped parsley

to taste, and fry it a few more minutes. In a bowl, we are going to pour the eggs and beat them until obtaining a homogeneous mixture.

3. Then in the pan where we have the sausage and broccoli fried, we are going to pour the eggs and let them cook for a few minutes. When we observe that the tortilla is almost done, we remove it carefully from the pan, we take it off and turn it so that it is cooked on the other side for a few more minutes.

4. Once the tortilla is ready we serve it and on top of it, we are going to put the sliced avocado, in addition, if it is of our taste we can sprinkle over it a little salt and pepper to give the final touch.

Chapter 17:
Sweet tooths, snacks and desserts

When starting any diet and mainly the Keto diet, we could feel hungry or anxious at some moments. To avoid that feeling it is advisable to eat some snacks as long as they are carbohydrates-free. This way we can stay in the Keto line. Let's remember that snacks are mostly a type of light food that we eat when we have anxiety, these in a certain way give us energy. The problem occurs when these snacks are eaten in large quantities and very often, as they are made from heavy ingredients that provide more fat to our body.

There are many ways to calm the anxiety or feeling of hunger with pleasant and healthy options so that we have are not guilty of giving us a taste. Next, we are going to show you a variety of options of snacks approved by experts in keto that will keep us satisfied without leaving the diet.

These recipes could be ideal as a snack or even as a dinner since they do not require much preparation:

- Slice of cheese spread with butter
- Celery stuffed with cream cheese
- Slice of cold butter spread with peanut butter
- Lettuce or cucumber spread with mayonnaise
- Small radishes with butter
- Parmesan cheese fries with butter
- Cheese and salami slices rolled up
- Sliced bacon with peanut butter or butter
- A square of dark chocolate with butter
- One tablespoon of butter or coconut oil melted in tea or coffee

On the other hand, we have a list of snacks a little more elaborated and tasty for those moments of anxiety. Ketogenic snacks are a good option to keep us on the diet in case we feel hungry.

Eggplant French Fries

Ingredients:

- 2 eggplants
- 475 ml (250 g) ground almonds
- 1 tsp cayenne pepper
- Salt and black pepper to taste
- 2 eggs
- 2 tbsp. coconut oil spray

Preparation:

1. Preheat oven to 400°F (200°C).
2. Peel the eggplants and cut into chips. Add salt (a little) on all sides to prevent the eggplant from becoming bitter.
3. In a not very deep bowl, mix the ground almond, cayenne, and pepper, in another bowl add the eggs beating until frothy.
4. Pass the chopped eggplants through the almonds, through the eggs and again through the almonds.
5. Place the eggplants "potatoes" in a baking tray previously greased, sprinkle coconut oil on top.
6. Bake for 15 minutes or until golden brown and crispy.

Bacon And Cheddar Cheese Balls

These balls are not only delicious but also ketogenic, bacon and cheddar cheese are a perfect and delicious combination, here we leave the preparation:

Ingredients:
- 150 g bacon
- 1 tablespoon of butter
- 150 g (150 ml) cream cheese
- 150 g cheddar cheese
- 50 g butter (at room temperature)
- ½ tsp ground black pepper

Preparation:
1. Melt the butter and fry the bacon until golden brown.
2. Remove from the frying pan and let cool on absorbent paper.
3. Cut the bacon into small pieces and place them in a bowl.
4. In another bowl, mix the excess fat from the bacon with the rest of the ingredients.
5. Leave the mixture in the refrigerator for 15 minutes to harden the mixture.
6. Assemble the balls, pass them over the bacon and serve.

Spinach, Artichoke And Cream Cheese Dip

Ingredients:
- 1 cucumber, chopped into sticks
- 2 cups spinach
- 2 artichoke hearts
- 1 tsp cream cheese
- Grain salt

Preparation:

1. Cook the spinach with a little grain salt, drain and cool.
2. Chop the cucumbers and reserve
3. Chop the artichoke hearts into four, add them in a bowl with the spinach.
4. Add the cream cheese, seasoning and mixing everything.

Focaccia Bread With Garlic And Rosemary

Ingredients:
- 175 g (375 m) shredded mozzarella.
- 2 tbsp (30g) cream cheese.
- 1 tsp. white wine vinegar.
- 1 egg.
- 175 ml (100 g) ground almonds.
- ½ tsp of salt.
- ½ tsp garlic powder.
- 50 g butter at room temperature.
- 3 cloves garlic, finely chopped
- ½ teaspoon of sea salt
- ½ tsp fresh chopped rosemary

Preparation:
1. Preheat oven to 200 °C (400 °F)
2. Heat cream cheese and mozzarella cheese in a saucepan over medium heat (microwaves can also be used) and stir occasionally.
3. Add the rest of the ingredients and mix.
4. Flatten the dough to a round shape, no more than 20 cm above the baking paper.
5. Using a fork, make small holes, bake for 12 minutes or until golden brown, then remove and let cool.
6. Prepare a mixture with garlic, butter, salt and rosemary, spread on bread and place on a grill or grill
7. Leave for 7 minutes

Mexican-Style Sausages

Ingredients:
- ½ cup chopped onion
- ½ tomato
- 2 turkey sausages
- Chili
- Grain salt

Preparation:
1. Add onion in a pan over medium heat until translucent.
2. Add the chili together with the tomato chopped in cubes, season with salt.
3. Chop the sausages in slices and add the sauce, let cook and serve.

Lettuce Cubes With Prickly Pear Salad

Ingredients:
- Lettuce (4 firm leaves well washed)
- 2 prickly pears
- Grain salt
- ½ cup onion
- 1 tsp olive oil
- 1 tsp vinegar
- 1 tbsp. chopped coriander
- 1 small chili-tomato

Preparation:
1. In a refractory add the prickly pears in cubes and leave them overnight with salt in grain (well covered).
2. Next day drain and let dry
3. Cut the onion and tomato into cubes and add them to the nopales.
4. Add olive oil, chopped coriander, and vinegar.

5. Place the mixture on the lettuce

Prepared Olives

Ingredients:
- 1 lemon (juice)
- ¼ cup chopped onion
- 6 Kalamata olives, pitted and stuffed
- 2 tbsp soy sauce

Preparation:
1. Cook the onion in a frying pan until translucent.
2. Add the olives and sprinkle with the sauce and lemon.
3. Let cool and serve

Cauliflower Bits With Peanut Butter

Ingredients:
- 2 tbsp peanut butter
- coarse salt
- 1 tbsp olive oil
- 1 cauliflower

Preparation:
1. Preheat oven to 400°F (200°C)
2. Cut the cauliflower
3. On a tray with waxed paper, put the cauliflowers and add olive oil, season and bake until golden brown.
4. Remove from oven and spread peanut butter, bake for a couple more minutes.
5. Remove from oven, let cool and serve

Additionally, for those who need something fast due to their short time due to work or travel, there are adequate snacks to the keto diet, among the most prominent are:

- Packaged olives (green, black or assorted)
- Beef bar (shredded pork or chicken sriracha)
- Cooked bacon
- Salami snacks
- Pork cracklings
- Macadamia nuts
- Pili nuts
- Very dark chocolate

Chard Skewers With Ham And Cheese

Ingredients:
- 3 thin slices of cooked ham
- 3 thin slices of cheese
- 3 leaves of chard well cleaned
- 2 large tomatoes, well washed

Preparation:
Cook the chard for a maximum time of 2 minutes, take it out of the water and then let it cool until it can be manipulated. Then, place it on a tray or plate and put on it the slices of ham and cheese carefully to avoid breaking the chards and roll them up. We chop in rolls and we take out three portions to assemble the skewer placing in each end a cube of tomato, then to serve. This recipe of skewers is perfect to consume between meals as a salty snack, however for the one that prefers, it can be a recipe for a dinner rich in proteins.

Crackers Of Crunchy Seeds And Oats

Ingredients:

- 20 grams of poppy seeds
- 20 grams of linseed
- 25 grams of chia seeds
- 55 grams of sesame seed
- 55 grams of pumpkin seeds
- 20 grams of thin layers of oats
- ¼ of caraway seeds
- ¼ teaspoon of granulated garlic or a clove of grated garlic
- 250ml of water

Preparation:

Turn on the oven at 150°C, place all the ingredients in a container except for the water, mix them all very well, add the water stirring little by little until it integrates with all the ingredients, leave to rest well covered for 10 minutes. After the time has elapsed, check that the water has been absorbed by the seeds. Its consistency should be a sticky dough where not even a drop should be left, otherwise, add a little oatmeal or chia, mix and wait again.

Place in the tray greased paper and then flatten using a roller or a kitchen spatula, the mixture should not be more than 3 to 5mm thick, put in the oven for a time of 30 to 35 minutes. After that time, with the spatula, introduce underneath the mixture, trying to turn very carefully to prevent it from breaking (you can use board or large plate), bake again for 25 to 30 minutes more, be careful to avoid burning. Remove from the oven, wait for it to cool down, cut on a board and cut with a good knife into pieces.

Chapter 18:
Keto drinks

As well as the Keto diet offers us varieties in sweet tooths and snacks to be consumed without any remorse, it also provides us different drinks and smoothies that are allowed and are within the ketogenic standards. Here we show you the different options so that you can choose according to your preference:

Keto Smoothie Chocolate

Have a necessary quantity of zucchini, coconut milk, and lettuce at your disposal. Romana, chia seeds, spinach, cocoa powder, avocado, sweetener of Passion fruit and mix everything to obtain a rich and sweet drink.

Chia seeds with blueberries and coconut

- 1 cup cashew or almond milk
- 2 tbsp. coconut oil
- 2 tbsp. ground chia seeds
- Sweetener equivalent to 2 tablespoons of sugar
- 1 cup blueberries
- 1 cup Greek yogurt (can be substituted for coconut milk without milk)
- ½ cup coconut

Mix all ingredients

Smoothie For Breakfast

It is a rich cocktail ideal to start the day based on the following ingredients: Spinach, coconut milk, greens powder, whey protein, almonds, Brazil nuts, spinach, sweet potato starch, and psyllium seeds; optionally, you can add some almonds to give a greater nutty flavor, then mix all the ingredients together and you'll get a nutritious drink to start the day.

Green shake

You only need the necessary amount of lemon, cucumber, avocado, and kale, all this is mixed with water, then blended and ready, is a rich and healthy drink

Smoothie with almond milk

This drink apart from being rich and healthy provides nutrients needed to start the day, you will only need celery, cucumber, matcha, spinach, avocado, and almond milk, then mix all the ingredients and finally, we add the chia seeds and coconut oil

Chia shake

This drink provides us with fiber

Ingredients:
- 1 tbsp walnut butter
- 1 tablespoon of chia seeds (soaked in water for 10 minutes)
- ¼ cup coconut milk
- 1 avocado
- 2 tsp. cocoa beans (if you want to add more flavor)
- 1 tsp. cocoa powder
- 1 scoop of chocolate protein powder
- 1 tbsp coconut oil

Blend all the ingredients mixing uniformly. If it is too thick, you can add 1 cup of water. At the moment of serving you can decorate with cocoa beans and cinnamon.

Green milkshake (without dairy products)

It is called green milkshake because it is the predominant color, the ingredients to use are avocado, kiwi, fresh ginger, fresh parsley, raw cucumber, fresh pineapple, and lettuce. We blend all the ingredients with water and we sweeten with any sugar substitute that is to your liking and preference.

Smoothie with macadamia nut oil

To prepare this shake you only need to mix avocado, spinach, stevia, coconut milk, cream, macadamia nut oil, vanilla protein, and oil of avocado, if you don't want to add or you don't have avocado oil at your disposal it can be replaced by olive oil or peanut oil.

Milkshake of almonds and blueberries

What it is necessary to achieve this tasty and nutrient-rich drink is to combine sugar-free almond sugar, a small amount of blueberries preferably organic, almond butter (it must be raw) and MCT oil

Strawberry milkshake

To achieve an excellent blend and obtain this smoothie it is necessary:
- 1 cup of fresh strawberries
- 1 tsp vanilla extract
- 1 tbsp coconut oil (you can also use any other healthy oil)
- 450ml coconut milk, if not available can be replaced by a cup of Greek yogurt if you prefer a milkshake (add water if it's too thick).

Raspberry vanilla smoothie

Ingredients:
- ½ cup natural strawberries (can be frozen)
- ½ cup unsweetened coconut milk
- 2/3 cup water
- ½ vanilla tsp (extract)

Then mix all the ingredients in the blender

Beet Smoothie

Mix in the blender the following ingredients to enjoy a delicious smoothie.

- 1 tbsp coconut oil
- 1 tbsp whey protein
- 1 tsp powdered cinnamon
- 1 cup almond milk, coconut milk can also be used
- 1 tbsp powdered beet

Walnut Smoothie:

- 1 pinch of salt
- 1 tsp powdered cinnamon
- 1 tablespoon peanut butter or cashew butter
- 2 tbsp preferably ground flax seeds
- 2 tbsp peeled walnuts
- 1 cup almonds

Combine all ingredients and blend

Ginger Smoothie

- Ingredients for its preparation:
- 30g frozen spinach
- 2 tbsp lemon juice
- 150ml of water
- 2 tsp. fresh stuffed ginger
- 75ml coconut cream or coconut milk

Combine all ingredients, add tablespoons of lemon one at a time. one to achieve the desired taste, after serving the drink we add a little of grated ginger and sprinkle over it.

Ketogenic coffee with cinnamon

This drink is ideal for those cold days, to make it you will need the following ingredients:

- 1 tsp ground cinnamon

- 475ml of water
- 2 tbsp ground coffee
- 75ml whipping cream

We combine the coffee with the cinnamon. We add the water and make it like coffee is normally made. Beat the cream with the help of a mixer until you get a mixture to point of snow, we serve in a large cup the coffee, add the whipped cream over it and finally add the cinnamon.

Chai tea

It is a warm and aromatic drink perfect for cold and rainy days.

Ingredients:
- 475ml of water
- 75ml whipping cream
- 1 tbsp chai tea

Follow the instructions on the chai tea container (hot water and tea), in the microwave, heat the cream in a medium cup and add the tea.

Coffee with pumpkinspices

Ingredients:
- ½ Tbsp vanilla extract
- 1 tbsp (25g) erythritol
- 1 tsp. spice mix for pumpkin pie
- 60ml (60g) pumpkin puree
- 60ml decaffeinated espresso coffee can also be strong coffee
- 225ml hot, unsweetened almond milk

Preparation:

Add all the ingredients in a blender and blend until a soft mixture is obtained, try it and give it the taste according to your preference, finally serve it.

Eggnog

Ingredients:
- ¼ honey tsp
- 1 pinch of ground nutmeg
- 225ml whipping cream
- 1 orange, the zest, and the juice
- 4 tbsp. brandy or any dark liqueur
- ¼ Tbsp vanilla extract

Preperation:
1. Mix the honey, vanilla powder and beaten egg yolks until the mixture is smooth, add ¼ of orange. Then we add 4 tablespoons of juice of orange, with the liqueur, carefully mix the whipping cream and combine it in a bowl with the egg mixture.
2. Serve in glasses and take to the refrigerator for 15 minutes.
3. This helps to develop more flavor and consistency in the eggnog

Flavored water

The cold flavored water refreshes when we feel like something without the need of adding calories Ingredients:
- 1 liter of cold, freshwater
- Flavorings of your free choice that can be fresh mint, cucumber or raspberries
- 475ml of ice

Preparation
1- Add the cold water in a pitcher
2- Place the chosen flavor and take it to the refrigerator leaving it to rest for at least 30 minutes
3- Fresh mint, citrus fruits such as orange, lemon or berries can be added if desired
4- With only a few slices are enough to give a rich flavor

Cold coffee

To soothe the heat, this delicious iced drink is an excellent choice.

Ingredients:
- 60ml whipping cream
- 225ml of coffee
- Ice cubes
- Vanilla extract (optional)

Instructions
1- As usual prepare the coffee, but twice as usual and leave it to cool down.
2- In a large glass add the ice cubes, add the coffee and then the cream.
3- Serve

Coffee with ketogenic cream

Ingredients:
- 60ml whipping cream
- 180ml of coffee

Preparation:
1- Choose the coffee of your preference and prepare it as usual.
2- In a small pot add the cream and heat, stir gently until it becomes frothy
3- In a large cup, pour the hot cream, add the coffee and stir
4- Serve instantly accompanied by a handful of yummy walnuts.

Keto Cheesecake

Ingredients:
- 2 passion fruit
- 2 tablespoons ricotta cheese
- 1 sachet of stevia
- 1 glass almond milk
- ice to taste

Preparation:

Add all the ingredients in a blender, mix everything and you're done. This way we'll get a delicious drink.

Chapter 19: 7 Day Meal Plan:

The 7-day meal plan aims to give a general idea of how the ketogenic diet might work effectively, however it is important to remember that it may work differently in each body.

This plan is based on a diet high in fat, low in carbohydrates and moderate in protein on which we could base the first week of our keto diet, however, we can refer to previous chapters for more recipes.

Monday

Breakfast: 2 sausages rolled in turkey with feta cheese and green tea
Snack: keto chocolate cheesecake
Lunch: Chicken Salad
Snack: pork rinds
Dinner: steamed vegetables and salmon

Tuesday

Breakfast: Cheese and mushroom omelet
Snack: Coffee without sugar
Lunch: Mexican Chicken Tacos
Snack: squares of ham and cheese
Dinner: Shrimp brochettes with bacon and onion

Wednesday

Breakfast: 2 boiled eggs wrapped in bacon strips and avocado strips with green tea

Snack: Light gelatin

Lunch: Chicken breast stuffed with ham and cream cheese.

Snack: Celery sticks with guacamole

Dinner: chop suey

Thursday

Breakfast: Turkey sausage and blended protein with strawberries

Snack: 40 grams of peanuts

Lunch: Steamed broccoli with fish

Snack: Nuts

Dinner: Fish skewers with bell pepper

Friday

Breakfast: Keto waffles with egg, cheese, and bacon

Snack: Coffee

Lunch: Asian-style sauteed keto cabbage

snack: gelatine

dinner: ham and cheese rolls

Saturday

Breakfast: salmon and bell pepper omelet

Snack: Merey

Lunch: Keto Caprese Omelet

Snack: Keto Smoothie

Dinner: Beef wraps

Sunday

Breakfast: Low-carbohydrate banana waffles

Snack: keto chocolate cake

Lunch: Ketogenic Tex Mex Casserole

Snack: Coconut biscuits without oven

Dinner: Stuffed avocados with smoked salmon

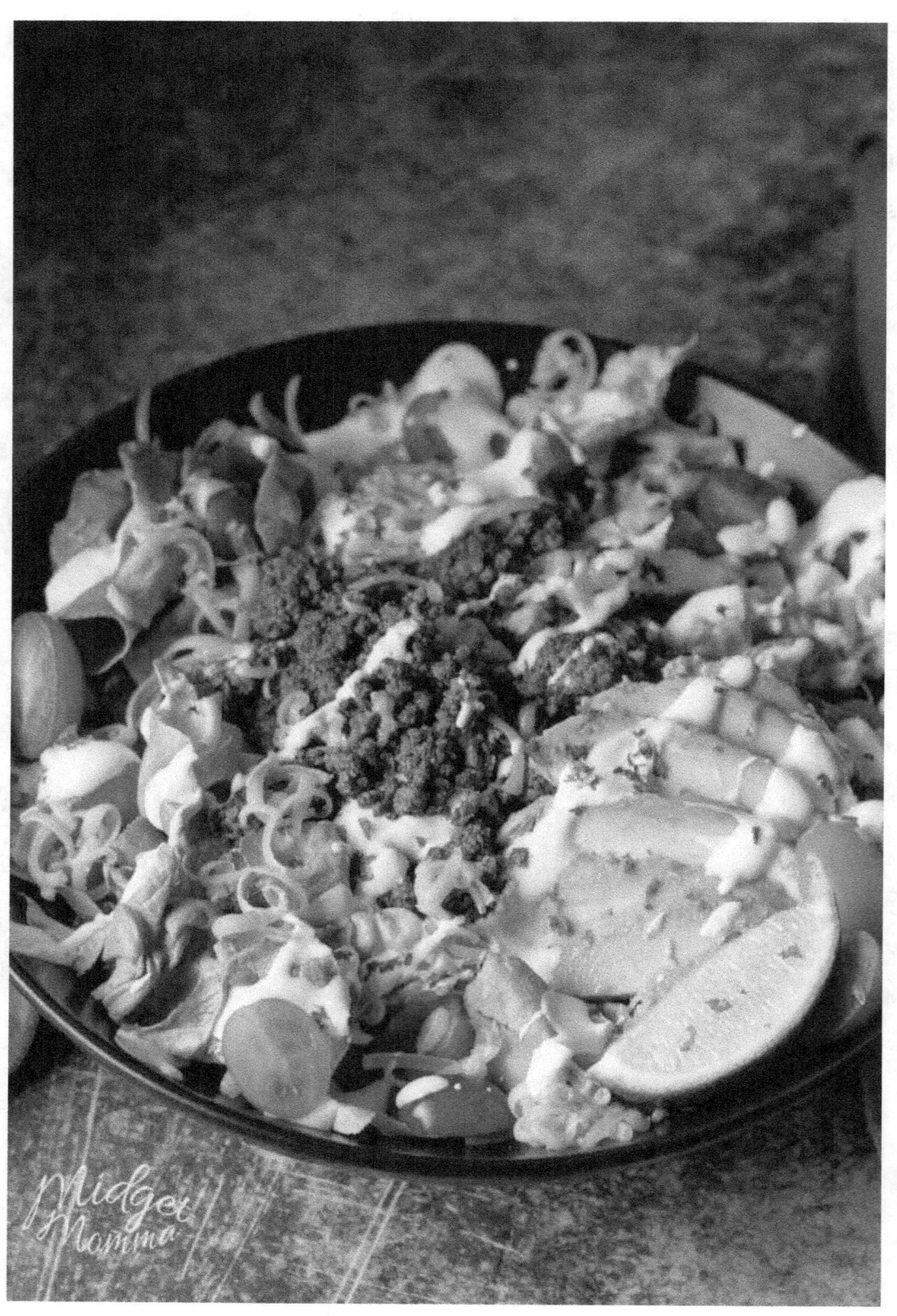

Conclusion

Thank you for making it through to the end of Keto for women: The ultimate beginners guide to know your food needs, weight loss, diabetes prevention and boundless energy with high-fat ketogenic diet recipes, let's hope it was informative and able to provide you with all of the tools you need to achieve your goals whatever they may be.

Now that you made it to the end of the book, you may know some, not to say all, of the benefits that the keto diet will have in your body. Even though it may be really hard to get started into this feeding plan, it absolutely worth it. Do not give up, fight for what you want, learn what your body needs and give it to it.

Women are known for being brave, amazing fighters and really strong so, are you going to let some extra pounds turn you down? As you could read, this diet is not only made for losing weight, there are studies that prove that this diet helps people who suffer from diabetes, decreases the symptoms of POS, helps in menstruation problems, improves brain and many other organs of our body.

Please, remember that even if you understood everything that is written in this book, and you feel like you can go keto on your own, it really recommended to go with a nutritionist or a specialist in the area for what you are using keto diet for. For example, if you are using keto to control POS, visit first your gyno.

Finally, if you found this book useful in any way, a review on Amazon is always appreciated!

Keto diet

An essential guide to begin a keto lifestyle With Quick & Easy Low-Carb Homemade Cooking

By

Sofia Wilson

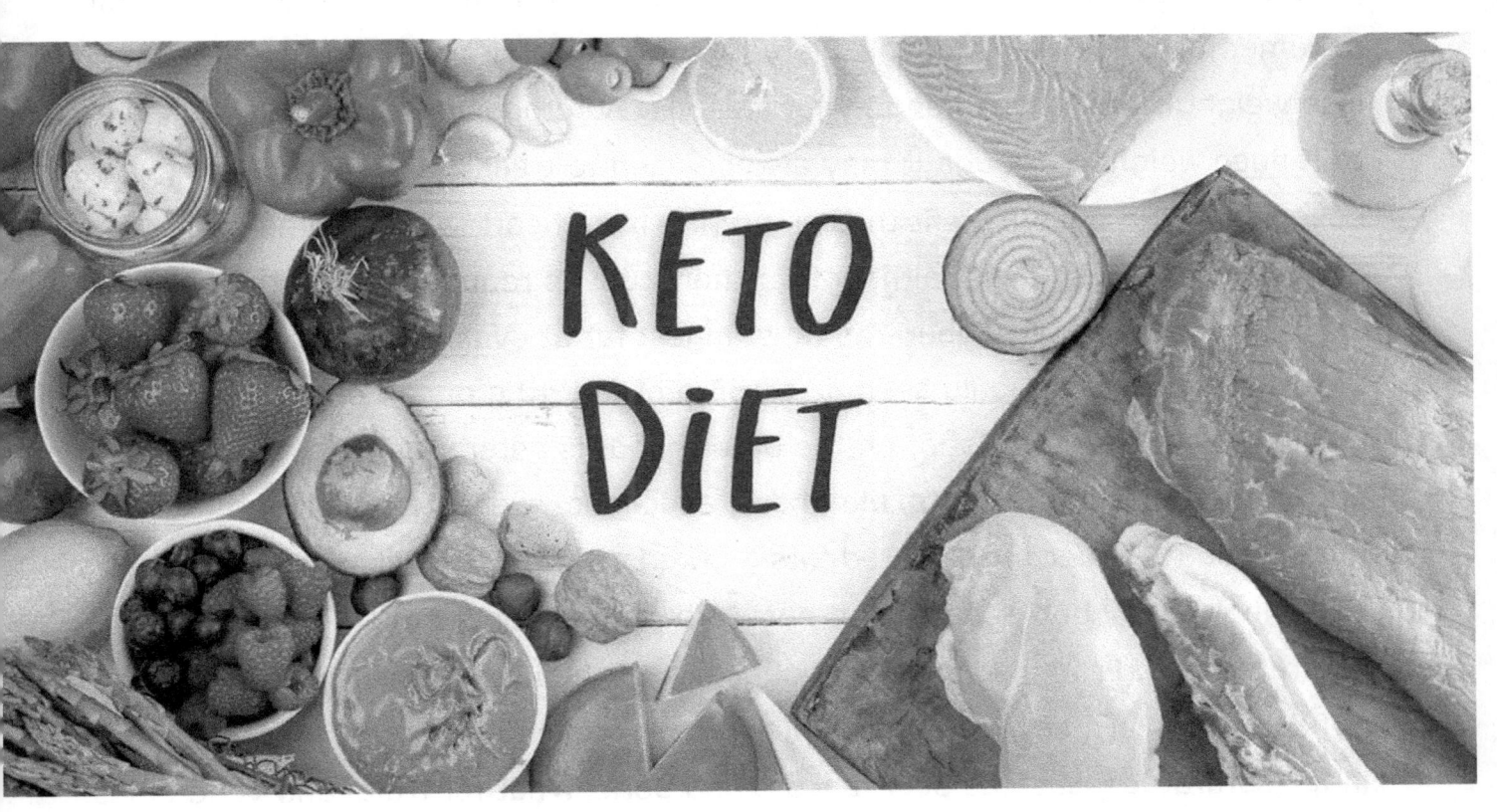

Introduction

Ketogenic refers to a low-carbohydrate diet. The aim is to eat more calories from fat and protein while eating fewer calories from carbohydrates. The carbohydrates that are easiest to digest, such as starch, pastries, soda, and white bread, are the first to go. When you consume fewer than 50 g of carbohydrates a day, your body easily runs out of energy. This normally takes three or four days. Then you'll begin to break down fat and protein for energy, potentially resulting in weight loss. Ketosis is the term for this state. It's crucial to remember that the ketogenic diet is a short-term diet designed to help you lose weight rather than change your lifestyle. A ketogenic diet is more often used to reduce weight, although it may also be used to treat medical problems such as epilepsy. It can even benefit those suffering from heart failure, some brain disorders, and even acne, although further study is required. Since the keto diet contains too much fat, adherents must ingest fat at every meal time. In a normal 2K-calorie diet, that would seem like 165 g of fat, 40 g of carbohydrates, and 75 g of protein. The exact ratio, on the other hand, is determined by your basic requirements. Nuts (walnuts, almonds), avocados, seeds, olive oil and tofu are among the healthier unsaturated fats allowed on the keto diet. However, oils (coconut, palm), butter, lard, and peanut butter all contain high amounts of saturated fats. Protein is an essential aspect of the keto diet, although it is also difficult to discern between protein items that are lean and protein products rich in fat(saturated), such as beef, bacon, and pork. What for fruits and vegetables? While fruits are generally rich in carbohydrates, unique fruits may be obtained in limited quantities (generally berries) Leafy greens (like kale, chard, Swiss chard, and spinach), broccoli, cauliflower, asparagus, tomatoes, brussels sprouts, bell peppers, garlic, cucumbers, mushrooms, summer squashes, as well as celery are also rich in carbohydrates. One cup of sliced broccoli includes about six carbohydrates. At the same time, there are several possible keto hazards, such as liver deficiency, liver complications, constipation, kidney disorders, and so on. As a result, we can also keep our Keto diet portions in check.

Understanding The Ketogenic Diet

This chapter delves into the Ketogenic diet in depth. The chapter further discusses which foods to consume on the Keto diet and which foods to stop while on this diet. The Keto diet is often explained in-depth, including how it functions and what health advantages it provides.

The ketogenic diet (or keto diet) is a high-fat, low-carbohydrate diet with various health benefits. Evidently, more than 20 studies suggest that this form of diet will help you lose weight and boost your wellbeing. Diabetes patients, epilepsy patients, patients suffering from Alzheimer's disease, as well as cancer can all benefit from ketogenic diets.

1.1 What is Keto?

The ketogenic diet is a very low carbohydrate, high-fat diet that has a lot in common with the Atkins diet and other low-carb diets. It necessitates a significant reduction of carbohydrate consumption and a replacement with fat. This reduction of carbohydrates puts the body into a metabolic condition known as ketosis. As this occurs, the body's energy production of fat-burning skyrockets. In addition, it converts fat into ketones in the liver, which will supply energy to the brain. Ketogenic diets can result in substantial reductions in insulin as well as blood sugar levels. This, along with the increased ketones, has numerous health benefits.

Ketogenic Diets Come in Many Forms
There are a few variations of the ketogenic diet, including:
The traditional ketogenic diet consists of a diet that is low in carbs, mild in protein, and strong in fats. It usually has a 75 percent fat content, a 5% carbohydrate content, and a 20% protein content.

The cyclic ketogenic diet entails high-carb reefed cycles, such as five ketogenic days accompanied by two days of high carbohydrate use.

A ketogenic diet with particular goals: The diet requires carbs to be inserted in between exercises.

Protein-rich ketogenic diet: This is comparable to a normal keto diet, but it contains extra protein. Usually, the ratio is 60 percent fat, 5% sugars, and 35 percent protein.

However, only normal and protein-rich ketogenic diets have been extensively studied. More complex keto diets, such as targeted or cyclic keto, are mainly utilized by bodybuilders and athletes.

Ketogenic Diet Health Benefits

In fact, the keto diet first gained popularity as a means of treating neurological conditions, such as epilepsy. Following that, research has shown that diet can help with a broad variety of health issues:

Heart disease: The keto diet has been found to decrease risk factors such as body fat, blood sugar, HDL cholesterol and blood pressure.

Alzheimer's disease: The ketogenic diet can ease Alzheimer's symptoms while still delaying the disease's progression.

Epilepsy: Research has demonstrated that a ketogenic diet can significantly reduce seizures in children with epileptic seizures.

Cancer: The diet is actually being used to control a number of diseases and to delay tumor development.

Acne: Lower insulin levels, as well as less sugar or fried food diets, will aid acne recovery.

Parkinson's disease: According to one report, diet can help relieve the effects of Parkinson's disease.

Brain injuries: One study found that the diet would also increase concussions and improve recovery after a brain injury.

Polycystic ovary syndrome: A ketogenic diet may help lower insulin levels and can be helpful in the treatment of polycystic ovary syndrome.

What foods can you consume on a ketogenic diet?

The majority of your meals will revolve around the following foods:
- Salmon, mackerel and tuna are representations of fatty fish.
- Look for pastured eggs, whole eggs, or omega-3 eggs.
- Seek for grass-fed butter plus cream wherever possible.
- Red meat, ham, sausage, turkey, bacon, chicken and steak are all examples of meat.
- Non-processed cheese (goat, cheddar, mozzarella, blue, or cream).
- Flax seeds, walnuts, almonds, pumpkin seeds, chia seeds and other nuts and beans
- Avocado oil, olive oil and coconut oil are the other safe oils.
- Salt, spices and pepper, as well as a variety of herbs, may be used as condiments.
- Avocados: entire avocados or guacamole made freshly.
- Low-carb vegetables including greens, tomatoes, onions, peppers and other related veggies.

Foods to avoid on a ketogenic diet include:

Carbohydrate-rich diets can be avoided as much as possible.

The following is a selection of items that must be eliminated or reduced on a ketogenic diet:
- Sugary drink, ice cream, soda, smoothies, cake, candy and other sugary items
- Wheat, pasta, cereals, rice, and other wheat-based products are examples of starches or grains.
- Sweet potatoes, parsnips, parsnips, potatoes, carrots and other tubers & root vegetables
- Reduced-calorie or low-fat foods are extremely processed and abundant in carbohydrates.
- Fruit: All fruits, with the exception of tiny bits of berries like strawberries.
- Chickpeas, lentils, peas, kidney beans, and other legumes or beans

- Some sauces/condiments: They are also high in unhealthy fat and sugar.
- Unhealthy fats: Limit the intake to mayonnaise, processed vegetable oils, and other processed fats.
- Alcohol: Because of their carb content, certain alcoholic beverages will shake you out of ketosis.
- Dietary ingredients that are sugar-free: Alcohols, which are often rich in sugar, may influence ketone levels in certain situations. These objects seem to have passed through a lot of refining as well.

1.2 What is the Keto diet, and how does it work?

The "ketogenic" keto diet consists of consuming a moderate level of protein, a heavy amount of fat, and relatively little carbohydrates; also, the fruit is forbidden. As for every diet fad, the advantages to adherents include improved vitality, weight reduction, and mental clarity. Is the ketogenic diet, though, what it's cracked up to be?

Dietitians and nutritionists are quiet on the topic. Low-carb diets like keto appear to assist with weight loss in the short term, but they are no more successful than any other self-help or conventional diet. They still don't seem to be enhancing athletic results.

The ketogenic diet was created to treat epilepsy instead of losing weight. In the 1920s, physicians found that holding people on low-carb diets induced their bodies to use fat as the predominant fuel source rather than glucose. When only fat is available for the body to combust or burn, the body converts fats to fatty acids, which are then converted to ketones, which can be used and taken up to power the body's cells.

Currently, feeding the body exclusively ketones prevents epilepsy for unclear causes. However, with the advent of anti-seizure medicines, few patients with epilepsy rely on ketogenic diets anymore, while certain people who may not respond to medications may benefit. Low carb diets like the Atkins diet, which gained popularity in the early 2000s, also spawned keto diets for weight loss. In comparison, all groups of meatier-meal diets restrict carbohydrates. This diet does not have a set structure, although most routines provide for fewer than fifty grams of carbs per day.

A keto diet causes the body to enter a state known as ketosis, in which the body's cells become completely reliant on ketones for nutrition. It's not exactly clear that this leads to weight loss, but ketosis decreases appetite and can affect hunger-controlling hormones, including insulin. As a consequence, proteins and fats can keep humans fuller longer than sugars, resulting in lower net calorie intake.

In one head-to-head comparison, researchers looked at 48 separate diet trials in which subjects were randomly allocated to one of the well-known diets. Low-carb diets like South Beach, Atkins, and Zone, as well as low-fat diets like Ornish diets and portion restriction diets like Weight Watchers and Jenny Craig, were among the options.

Every diet resulted in greater weight loss than almost no diet after six months, according to the results. Low-carb and low-fat dieters lost almost equal amounts of weight as compared to non-dieters, with low-carb dieters losing 19 pounds on average versus low-fat dieters dropping 17.6 pounds (7.99 kilograms). At 12 months, both diet styles displayed symptoms of dropping off, with low-fat and low-carb dieters being 16 pounds (7.27 kg) smaller on average than non-dieters.

There were few differences in weight reduction within the diets of designated people. This is in line with the practice of recommending every diet that an individual practice in order to lose weight.

Another study of well-known diets discovered the Atkins diet, which results in greater weight loss than merely teaching people about portion control. Nevertheless, several of the scientific researched about this low-carb diet featured licensed dietitians assisting respondents in making food decisions, rather than the self-directed approach used by most people. This has been seen in other diet studies, according to the researchers, and the tests' results seem to be more positive in the real world than the weight loss.

Finally, a simple comparison between low-carb versus low-fat dieting revealed that there was a statistically significant difference in the amount of weight lost over a year. Low-carbohydrate dieters dropped an average of 13 pounds (6 kg), compared to 11.7 pounds for low-fat dieters (5.3 kg).

Ketogenic diets may help us lose weight, but they are no more successful than other diet methods. Since carbohydrate reserves in the body comprise water molecules, the bulk of the weight lost during the early stages of a ketogenic diet is water weight. This gives the scale an exciting amount at first, but weight reduction slows down with time.

What are the keto effects, and how can they help?

The advantages of a keto diet are close to that of other high-fat, low-carb diets, but it tends to be more successful than centrist low-carb diets. Keto is a low-carb, high-fat diet that maximizes health benefits. However, it will slightly raise the likelihood of complications.

Aid in weight loss

Weight reduction can be improved by converting the body into a fat-burning device. Insulin levels – the hormone that retains fat – are falling rapidly, suggesting that fat burning has risen dramatically. This seems to make it much easier to lose bodyweight without going hungry.

More than thirty high-quality observational studies show that low-carb and keto diets are more effective than other diets at losing weight.

Reverse type 2 diabetes by regulating blood sugar

A ketogenic diet has been shown in research to be successful in the treatment of type 2 diabetes, with total disease reversal occurring in certain instances. It makes perfect sense since keto removes the need for therapy, lowers blood sugar levels, and eliminates the potential negative consequences of high insulin levels.

Since a keto diet will reverse type 2 diabetes, it is likely to be helpful in preventing and reversing pre-diabetes. Keep in mind that "reversal" in this context refers to changing the disease, improving glucose tolerance, and reducing the need for care. It may be so drastically altered that after therapy, blood pressure returns to normal with time. In this context, reversal refers to progressing or deteriorating in the reverse direction of the condition. Changes in your lifestyle, on the other side, just succeed if you bring them into effect. If a person returns to the way of life he or she has before diabetes type 2 appeared and advanced, it is possible that success would return with time.

Improve your mental and physical performance:
Some people use ketogenic diets to boost their mental performance. It's also normal for people to feel more energized while they're in ketosis.
They don't need nutritional carbs for the brain on keto. It runs on ketones 24 hours a day, seven days a week, with a small amount of glucose synthesized in the liver. Carbohydrates are not necessary for the diet. As a result, ketosis leads to a steady flow of food (ketones) to the brain, avoiding significant blood sugar spikes. This will also assist with improved focus and attention, as well as clearing brain fog and improving mental awareness.

Epilepsy Treatment

The keto diet has been used to manage epilepsy since the 19th and 20th centuries and has proved to be effective. It has historically been used mainly for adolescents, although in recent years, it has also proved to be useful to adults. Or, used in conjunction with a keto diet, certain people with epilepsy might be able to take less to no anti-epileptic drugs while being seizure-free. This may help to reduce the drug's adverse effects while still improving cognitive capacity.

Breakfast, Lunch and Dinner Recipes

1 Hot Chocolate

(Ready in about 10 minutes | Serving 1 | Difficulty: Easy)

Per serving: Kcal 173, Fat: 17g, Net Carbs: 5g, Protein: 3g

Ingredients

- 2 tbsp cocoa powder, unsweetened, plus extra for garnish
- 1/4 tsp. of vanilla extract
- 1 1/4 cup of water
- 2 1/2 tsp of keto sugar
- 1/4 cup of heavy cream
- Whipped cream

Instructions

Add cocoa and sugar to a frying pan over moderate flame and whisk. Add 2tbsp water and increase the flame. Add rest of water plus cream and whisk frequently. Add vanilla and stir. Pour mixture in mug and top with whipped cream. Sprinkle cocoa powder and enjoy.

2 Classic bacon with eggs

(Ready in about 10 minutes | Serving 4 | Difficulty: Easy)

Per serving: Kcal 425, Fat: 31g, Net Carbs: 2g, Protein: 33g

Ingredients

- 8 eggs
- cherry tomatoes
- 9 oz. bacon, sliced
- fresh thyme

Instructions

Add bacon to the pan and fry over moderate flame. Add to the plate once it turns crispy and place aside. Fry eggs in the fat left in the pan. Cook to your preference and add tomatoes and cook as well. Add pepper and salt and eat with bacon.

3 keto breakfast

(Ready in about 10 minutes | Serving 1 | Difficulty: Easy)

Per serving: Kcal 424, Fat: 41g, Net Carbs: 1g, Protein: 13g

Ingredients

- 1 cup of baby spinach
- 2 eggs
- 2 tbsp of mayonnaise
- 1 tbsp of butter
- black pepper and salt

Instructions

Warm butter in a pan over moderate flame and add cracked eggs. Cook eggs according to your preference and add pepper and salt over them. Serve with a dollop of mayonnaise plus baby spinach. Have a cup of black coffee along.

4 Spinach and scrambled eggs

(Ready in about 8 minutes | Serving 1 | Difficulty: Easy)

Per serving: Kcal 368, Fat: 32g, Net Carbs: 2g, Protein: 18g

Ingredients

- 1 tbsp of butter
- black pepper and salt
- 2 eggs
- 2 tbsp of whipping cream
- 1 cup of baby spinach
- 1 oz. salmon smoked

Instructions

Warm butter in a pan over moderate flame and fry baby spinach until it turns soft. Add cream and cook until it bubbles and turns creamy. Breaks eggs into the pan and mix to incorporate all the ingredients. Season using pepper and salt. Continue stirring and cook according to your preference. Add eggs to the pan and serve with smoked salmon.

5 Oven pancake

(Ready in about 40 minutes | Serving 4 | Difficulty: Moderate)

Per serving: Kcal 553, Fat: 49g, Net Carbs: 5g, Protein: 22g

Ingredients

- 31/2 oz. pork bacon
- 2 tbsp of butter 4 eggs
- 1 tsp of baking powder
- 2 oz. of yellow onion
- 1 cup of whipping cream
- 1/2 cup of almond flour
- 1/2 cup cottage cheese
- 1 tbsp of husk powder
- 1 tsp of salt

Instructions

Preheat the oven to 350 degrees F. Dice onion and bacon. Warm butter in a pan and cook onion and bacon in the pan until the bacon gets crispy and onion is translucent. Add the rest of the ingredients to a bowl and mix. Pour mixture in a pan and top with onions and bacon. Bake for around 25 minutes and enjoy.

6 Pulled Pork

(Ready in about 20 minutes | Serving 1 | Difficulty: Easy)

Per serving: Kcal 153, Fat: 10, Net Carbs: 8g, Protein: 6g

Ingredients

- 2 tbsp of olive oil
- 1/4 tsp of salt
- 2 eggs
- 1 (115g) diced turnip 1/2 tsp paprika
- 1/4 tsp of garlic powder
- 3 halved(50g) Brussels sprouts
- 1/4 tsp of black pepper
- 1 cup of spinach chopped
- 3 ounces of pulled pork
- 2 tbsp diced red onion
- 1 tbsp of parsley chopped

Instructions

Warm oil in a pan over moderate flame. Add spices and turnip and cook for around 5 minutes.

Add the rest of the veggies and cook for around 3 minutes. Add pork and cook for 2 more minutes. Break eggs and cook for around 5 minutes, covered. Season using pepper and salt and top with parsley.

7 Bacon Egg Cups

(Ready in about 30 minutes | Serving 12 | Difficulty: Easy)

Per serving: Kcal 115, Fat: 8g, Net Carbs: 0g, Protein: 9g

Ingredients

- Bacon strips 12
- pepper, to taste
- 12 Big eggs

Instructions

Preheat the oven to 400 degrees F. Spray a muffin tin using cooking spray and place aside. Use one bacon piece for every muffin and form a basket for the egg. Add bacon inside in a way that it covers the sides, and use scissors to remove the extra bacon. Add this to the bottom of the basket and repeat with the rest of the bacon pieces. Bake for around 7 minutes and break an egg in each basket. Bake for another 15 minutes. Season using pepper and enjoy.

8 Granola Clusters

(Ready in about 45 minutes | Serving 8 | Difficulty: Moderate)

Per serving: Kcal 327, Fat: 31.5, Net Carbs: 6g, Protein: 5.5

Ingredients

- 1 cup of pecan halves
- 1/2 cup of almonds
- 1/4 cup of powdered Sweetener
- 1 cup of flaked coconut
- 1/2 cup of pumpkin seeds
- 1/2 cup of butter
- 1/2 tsp of salt
- 1/4 cup of Swerve Brown
- 1/2 tsp of vanilla extract

Instructions

Preheat the oven to 300 degrees F. Use parchment paper to line a baking dish. Combine everything except sweeteners and butter in a blender and blend. Add sweeteners and butter in a pan placed on low flame. Whish until sweeteners are dissolved, and butter melts. Add nut mixture and mix. Pour mixture in a prepared pan in a single layer. Top with parchment paper and bake for around 30 minutes.

9 Crustless Quiche

(Ready in about 35 minutes | Serving 6 | Difficulty: Moderate)

Per serving: Kcal 216, Fat: 17g, Net Carbs: 4g, Protein: 11g

Ingredients

- 1/2 cup of bacon chopped
- 1/4 tsp of black pepper ground
- 1/2 cup of chopped cherry tomatoes
- 1/2 cup of broccoli chopped
- 1/2 tsp of salt
- 1/2 cup of milk
- 2/3 cup mozzarella cheese shredded
- 1/2 cup of half and half
- 5 eggs

Instructions

Preheat the oven to 325 degrees F. Use cooking spray to spray a baking dish and spread tomatoes, broccoli, plus bacon evenly on the dish. Combine the rest of the ingredients in a bowl and pour over veggies. Sprinkle cheese on top and bake for around 25 minutes.

10 Fluffy Eggs

(Ready in about 10 minutes | Serving 4 | Difficulty: Easy)

Per serving: Kcal 281, Fat: 20.2g, Net Carbs: 5.2g, Protein: 19.7g

For Scrambled eggs

- 1 handful of chives
- Black pepper ground
- 4 ounces of goat cheese
- 8 eggs
- 1/2 tsp of kosher salt
- 2 tbsp of butter

Instructions

Dice the chives. Whisk eggs in a bowl and add goat cheese. Add pepper and salt and stir. Warm butter in a pan over moderate flame. Add eggs mixture, and once eggs start to harden, make folds with a spatula by slowly scraping egg sections. Garnish with chives and enjoy.

11 Keto Pancakes

(Ready in about 10 minutes | Serving 4 | Difficulty: Easy)

Per serving: Kcal 395, Fat: 34, Net Carbs: 12g, Protein: 14g

Ingredients

- 1 cup of almond flour
- 1/3 cup unsweetened almond milk
- 2-3 tbsp of sweetener of choice
- 1/4 tsp of salt
- 1/4 cup of coconut flour
- 5 large eggs
- 1 tsp of baking powder gluten-free
- 1 1/2 tsp of vanilla extract
- 1/4 cup of coconut oil
- Berries

Instructions

Add all the ingredients to a bowl and mix. Preheat the griddle to approximately 300 degrees F. Pour a quarter of the mixture onto the griddle and heat for around 2 minutes. Flip to cook the other side for 2 minutes as well. Repeat with the remaining mixture and enjoy.

12 Frittata Muffins

(Ready in about 30 minutes | Serving 12 | Difficulty: Easy)

Per serving: Kcal 164, Fat: 14g, Net Carbs: 4g, Protein: 7g

Ingredients

- 4 tbsp of avocado oil
- 3 minced garlic cloves
- 1/2 pound thawed frozen spinach squeezed dry
- 1/2 medium diced onion
- 1/2 pound sliced cremini mushrooms
- 5 ounces of Prosciutto di Parma
- Kosher salt
- 2 tbsp of coconut flour
- 8 Big eggs
- Ground pepper
- 1/4 cup of coconut milk
- 1 cup halved cherry tomatoes

Instructions

Preheat the oven to 375 degrees F. Warm 2 tbsp of avocado oil in a frying pan over moderate flame. Sauté onions until translucent. Add mushrooms and garlic and cook until the moisture from mushrooms evaporates. Season filling using pepper and salt. Transfer to a plate. Beat eggs with the rest of the ingredients in a separate bowl to prepare the batter. Add spinach and mushrooms and mix. Brush muffin tin with remaining avocado oil and use prosciutto to line all cups. Pour frittata batter in every cup and top with diced tomatoes. Bake for around 20 minutes and turn at half point.

13 Bacon Omelet

(Ready in about 32 minutes | Serving 4 | Difficulty: Easy)

Per serving: Kcal 311, Fat: 20g, Net Carbs: 3g, Protein: 17g

Ingredients

- 8 eggs
- 4 cooked bacon slices chopped
- 1 sliced leek
- 2 tbsp of ghee
- Micro greens
- Black pepper ground and sea salt
- Fresh minced chives

Instructions

Neat eggs in a bowl and season using pepper and salt. Melt ghee in a pan over moderate flame. Cook leek for around 5 minutes in the pan and add cooked bacon plus egg mixture in the pan. Cook until it starts to settle and flip to cook the other side for around 3 minutes. Top with chives and micro greens.

14 Brie Frittata

(Ready in about 25minutes | Serving 6 | Difficulty: Easy)

Per serving: Kcal 338, Fat: 27g, Net Carbs: 1.8g, Protein: 18g

Ingredients

- 8 slices chopped bacon
- 1/2 cup of whipping cream
- 8 Big eggs
- 2 minced cloves garlic
- 1/2 tsp of pepper
- 1/2 tsp of salt
- 4 ounces sliced brie

Instructions

Cook bacon in a pan until it turns crispy. Drain on a plate lined with a paper towel. Whisk eggs with the rest of the ingredients plus bacon(two-thirds). Pour mixture in a pan containing bacon grease and cook until egg at edges set up and is somewhat loose in the center. Layer the diced brie on eggs and sprinkle the rest of the bacon. Preheat the broiler to high temperature and position the oven rack in the oven at the second-highest point. Broil for around 5 minutes.

15 Fried Rice

(Ready in about 30 minutes | Serving 4 | Difficulty: Easy)

Per serving: Kcal 108, Fat: 7g, Net Carbs: 21g, Protein: 13g

Ingredients

- 1 diced into florets cauliflower head
- 1 sliced bunch of scallions
- 2 tbsp of coconut oil
- 3 minced garlic cloves
- 2 peeled carrots, diced
- 1 tbsp fresh ginger minced
- 2 diced celery stalks
- 1 cup of frozen peas
- 1 diced bell pepper
- 2 tbsp of rice vinegar
- 2 tsp of Sriracha
- 3 tbsp of soy sauce

Garnishes

- 1 tbsp coconut oil
- Black pepper ground and sea salt
- 4 tbsp scallions sliced
- 4 eggs
- 4 tbsp fresh cilantro chopped
- 4 tsp of sesame seeds

Instructions

Pulse cauliflower in food processor's bowl for around 3 minutes and place aside. Warm oil in a pan and add ginger, scallions and garlic and cook for around 1 minute. Add celery, bell pepper and carrots and cook for around 11 minutes. Add cauliflower rice and cook for 5 additional minutes. Add frozen peas and mix. Add sriracha, rice vinegar and soy sauce and mix. Place aside. Warm oil in a pan and break eggs in it. Cook for around 4 minutes and season using pepper and salt. Top rice with egg and garnish using 1 tbsp cilantro, tsp sesame seeds and 1 tbsp scallions in four plates.

16 Thai Soup

(Ready in about 22 minutes | Serving 6 | Difficulty: Easy)

Per serving: Kcal 323, Fat: 27g, Net Carbs: 7g, Protein: 15g

Ingredients

Main Soup

- 4 Boneless Chicken Thighs skin removed
- 2 tsp of Thai curry paste
- 4 cloves Garlic, crushed
- 14.5 oz of Coconut Milk
- 2 tsp of Fish Sauce
- 1 tsp of Agave nectar
- 3 tsp of Soy Sauce
- 2 Chopped Green Scallions
- 2 inches chopped Minced Ginger

Veggies

- 1/2 cup of sliced cherry tomatoes
- 3 chopped green scallions
- 1/4 cup of chopped cilantro
- 1 lime, juiced

Instructions

Add soup ingredients in an instant pot and close. Cook by pressing the soup button for around 12 minutes under pressure. Release pressure using quick technique and take out chicken shred and add back to the soup. Add vegetables to broth and sear.

17 Buffalo Soup

(Ready in about 30 minutes | Serving 6 | Difficulty: Easy)

Per serving: Kcal 270, Fat: 16g, Net Carbs: 4g, Protein: 27g

Ingredients

- 1/2 large diced Onion
- 1 tbsp Olive oil
- 1/2 cup diced Celery
- 1 lb cooked shredded chicken
- 4 minced cloves Garlic
- 4 cups of Chicken broth
- 6 oz cubed Cream cheese
- 3 tbsp of Buffalo sauce
- 1/2 cup of half & half

Instructions

Select sauté setting on the instant pot. Add celery, onion and oil. Cook for around 10 minutes. Add garlic and sauté for around one minute. Turn the pot off and add chicken, buffalo sauce and broth. Cover the pot and seal it. Select soup setting and adjust the timer to 5 minutes. After done, release pressure naturally for around 5 minutes and turn to instant release and take the lid off. Ladle around a cup of liquid from the pot and add to the blender without chicken. Add cream cheese and puree. Pour mixture into the pot and add half and half and stir.

18 Jalapeno Soup

(Ready in about 25minutes | Serving 4 | Difficulty: Easy)

Per serving: Kcal 446, Fat: 35g, Net Carbs: 4g, Protein: 28g

Ingredients

- 4 slices of bacon
- 1/2 diced medium onion
- 2 tbsp of butter
- 1/4 cup chopped pickled jalapenos
- 2 cups shredded chicken cooked
- 2 cups of chicken broth
- 4 ounces of cream cheese
- Pepper and salt
- 1 cup sharp cheddar shredded
- 1/3 cup of heavy cream
- 1/4 tsp of garlic powder

Instructions

Fry bacon in a pan until crispy and crumble it and place aside. In the meantime, place the pot over moderate flame and add onion and butter. Saute for around 2 minutes and add half amount of bacon and jalapenos. Add chicken and broth and boil. Then reduce the flame and simmer for around 20 minutes. Add cream cheese to a bowl and microwave for around 20 seconds. Stir and add to soup. Mix heavy cream as well. Add grated cheese and until it is melted, stir. Serve with the rest of the bacon on top.

19 Sausage with Peppers

(Ready in about 2 hours 5 minutes | Serving 6 | Difficulty: Hard)

Per serving: Kcal 313, Fat: 21.7g, Net Carbs: 14g, Protein: 16.4g

Ingredients

- 1 tbsp Olive oil
- 3 diced into strips Bell peppers
- 6 medium Pork links of sausages
- 1 sliced large Onion
- 1/2 tsp of Sea salt
- 1 tbsp of Italian seasoning
- 6 minced cloves Garlic
- 1/4 tsp of Black pepper
- 1 1/2 cups of Marinara sauce

Instructions

Warm oil in a pan over moderate flame. Add sausage and cook for around 2 minutes on each side. Add the rest of the ingredients except marinara in the meantime in a slow cooker. Toss to mix and spread the marinara sauce in a layer on veggies. Add sausage and cook for around 3 hours on a high setting.

20 Beef Barbacoa

(Ready in about 4 hours 10 minutes | Serving 9 | Difficulty: Hard)

Per serving: Kcal 242, Fat: 11g, Net Carbs: 2g, Protein: 32g

Ingredients

- 3 lb trimmed Beef brisket diced into chunks of 2 inch
- 2 Chipotle chiles in adobo medium
- 2 whole Bay leaf
- 1/2 cup of Beef broth
- 5 minced Garlic cloves
- 1 tbsp of Dried oregano
- 2 tbsp of Apple vinegar
- 2 tsp of Sea salt
- 2 tbsp of Lime juice
- 2 tsp of Cumin
- 1 tsp of Black pepper

Instructions

Add all the ingredients except beef plus bay leaves in a blender and puree. You will get a smooth mixture. Add beef to the slow cooker and pour blender mixture on it. Add bay leaves and cook for 6 hours at the high setting.

21 Cauliflower Shrimp

(Ready in about 30 minutes | Serving 2 | Difficulty: Easy)

Per serving: Kcal 302, Fat: 18g, Net Carbs: 13g, Protein: 24g

Spicy Shrimp

- 1 tbsp of paprika
- 1 pound deveined shrimp peeled
- 2 tsp of garlic powder
- 1 tbsp of olive oil
- 1/2tsp of cayenne pepper
- Black pepper ground and salt

Cauliflower Grits

- 1 tbsp of unsalted butter
- 1 cup of whole milk
- 4 cups of riced cauliflower
- 1/2 cup of crumbled goat cheese
- Black pepper ground and salt

Garlic Arugula

- 1 tbsp of extra-virgin olive oil
- 4 cups of baby arugula
- 3 sliced garlic cloves
- Black pepper ground and salt

Instructions

Mix cayenne, paprika and garlic powder in a bowl. Add shrimp to a sealable bag and add the mixture in it. Toss and refrigerate the bag. Melt butter in a pot over moderate flame. Cook cauliflower rice for around 3minutes. Add half amount of milk and simmer for around 8 minutes. Add rest of milk and simmer for around 10 minutes. Add goat cheese and season using pepper and salt. Warm 1 tbsp oil in a pan for garlic arugula. Sauté garlic for around 1 minute. Add arugula and sauté for

around 4minutes. Season using pepper and salt and take out on a plate. Add the rest of the olive oil in this pan and sauté shrimp for around 5 minutes. Season using pepper and salt. Divide grits equally among 4 plates and top with a quarter amount of each shrimp and arugula.

22 Cheese Spinach

(Ready in about 10 minutes | Serving 4 | Difficulty: Easy)

Per serving: Kcal 166, Fat: 15.1, Net Carbs: 1.7, Protein: 4.4

Ingredients

- 1 tbsp butter, room temperature
- 1 clove garlic, minced
- 10 ounces spinach
- 1/2 tsp garlic salt
- 1/4 tsp ground black pepper, or more to taste
- 1/2tsp cayenne pepper
- 3 ounces cream cheese
- 1/2 cup double cream

Instructions

Add butter to a pan and melt over moderate flame. Cook garlic for around 30 seconds and add spinach. Cook for around 2 minutes, covered. Season with cayenne, pepper and salt. Add cream and cheese and cook until it melts.

23 Tangy Chicken Drumettes

(Ready in about 40 minutes | Serving 4 | Difficulty: Moderate)

Per serving: Kcal 209, Fat: 12.2g, Net Carbs: 0.4, Protein: 23.2g

Ingredients

- 1 pound chicken drumettes
- 1 tbsp olive oil
- 2 tbsp butter, melted
- 1garlic cloves, sliced
- Fresh juice of 1/2 lemon
- 2 tbsp white wine
- Salt and ground black pepper, to taste
- 1 tbsp fresh scallions, chopped

Instructions

Preheat the oven to 440 degrees F. Line a pan using parchment paper and add chicken. Drizzle with butter and oil. Add the rest of the ingredients and bake for around 35 minutes. Garnish with scallions.

24 Ranch Chicken

(Ready in about 20 minutes | Serving 4 | Difficulty: Easy)

Per serving: Kcal 295, Fat: 19.5g, Net Carbs: 2.9g, Protein: 3.1g

Ingredients

- 2 chicken breasts
- 2 tbsp butter, melted
- 1 tsp salt
- 1/2 tsp garlic powder
- 1/2 tsp cayenne pepper
- 1/2 tsp black peppercorns, crushed
- 1/2 tbsp ranch seasoning mix
- 4 ounces Ricotta cheese, room temperature
- 1/2 cup Monterey-Jack cheese, grated
- 4 slices bacon, chopped
- 1/4 cup scallions, chopped

Instructions

Preheat the oven to 370 degrees F. Drizzle butter over chicken. Add seasonings to chicken and cook chicken in the pan for around 5 minutes on each side. Coat a baking dish and add chicken. Add bacon and cheese and bake for around 12 minutes. Add scallions on top.

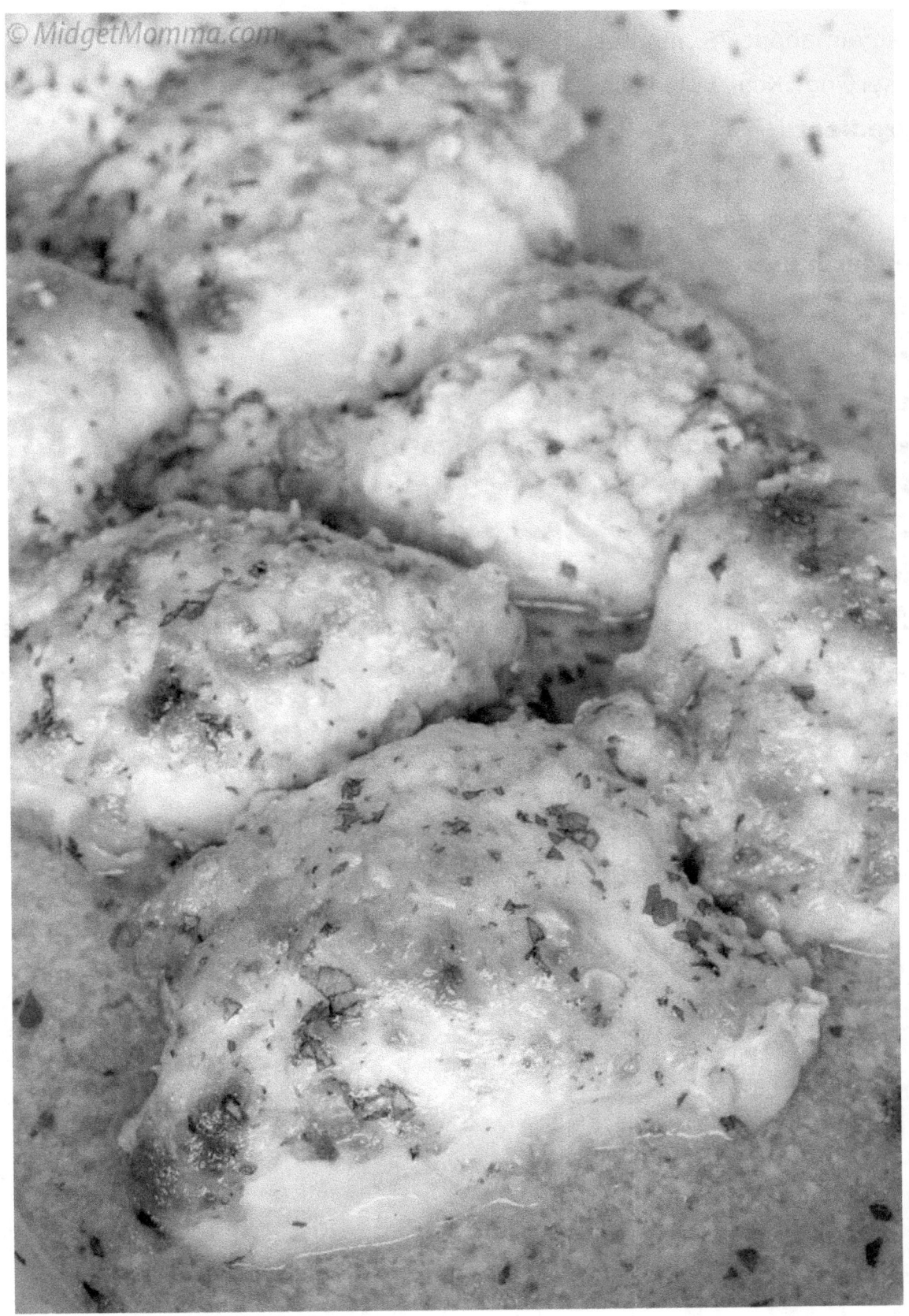

25 Garlic Chicken Wings

(Ready in about 25 minutes | Serving 4 | Difficulty: Easy)

Per serving: Kcal 131, Fat: 7.8g, Net Carbs: 1.8g, Protein: 13.4g

Ingredients

- 8 chicken wings
- 2 tbsp ghee, melted

The Marinade

- 2 garlic cloves, minced
- 1/4 cup leeks, chopped
- 2 tbsp lemon juice
- Salt and ground black pepper, to taste
- 1/2 tsp paprika
- 1 tsp dried rosemary

Instructions

Add marinade ingredients in a bowl and coat chicken with it. Cover and leave for around1 an hour. Preheat the grill to moderate temperature. Drizzle chicken with melted ghee and grill for around 20 minutes.

26 Steak Salad

(Ready in about 20 minutes | Serving 4 | Difficulty: Easy)

Per serving: Kcal 231, Fat: 17g, Net Carbs: 6g, Protein: 13.8g

Ingredients

- 2 tbsp olive oil
- 8 ounces flank steak, salt-and-pepper-seasoned
- 1 cucumber, sliced
- 1/2 cup onions, finely sliced
- 1 ripe avocado, peeled and sliced
- 2 medium-sized heirloom tomatoes, sliced
- 2 ounces baby arugula
- 1 tbsp fresh coriander, chopped
- 3 tbsp lime juice

Instructions

Warm 1 tbsp oil in a pan over moderate flame and cook steak for around 5 minutes. Transfer steak to bowl and add rest of ingredients. Drizzle the rest of the oil and lime juice and eat after chilling.

27 Catfish

(Ready in about 25 minutes | Serving 4 | Difficulty: Easy)

Per serving: Kcal 510, Fat: 40g, Net Carbs: 5.5g, Protein: 31.3g

Ingredients

- 1 tbsp of sesame oil
- 4 scallions
- 11 ounces of cauliflower
- 2 ounces of butter
- 1 minced garlic clove
- Black pepper ground and salt
- 1 tspgrated ginger root
- Cayenne pepper
- 1 sprig crushed rosemary
- 2 sprigs crushed dried thyme
- 24 ounces of catfish
- 1/2 cup of double cream
- 1/2 cup of cream cheese
- 1 egg

Instructions

Preheat the oven to around 390 degrees F. Spray casserole dish using cooking spray. Add oil to pan and warm over moderate flame. Cook scallions and cauliflower for around 5 minutes. Add ginger and garlic and cook for one more minute. Transfer veggies to the dish and sprinkle using seasonings. Top with catfish. Mix cream, cheese and egg in a bowl and spread over casserole. Add butter slices on top and bake for around 22 minutes.

28 Salad- Swedish Style

(Ready in about 8 minutes | Serving 3 | Difficulty: Easy)

Per serving: Kcal 134, Fat: 7.9g, Net Carbs: 5.4g, Protein: 10.2g

Ingredients

- 1/2 cup of baby spinach
- 6 ounces of flaked herring pieces pickled
- 2tbspof basil leaves
- 1 chopped bell pepper
- 2 tbspof chopped fresh chives
- Black pepper ground and salt
- 1 tsp of minced garlic
- 1 chopped red onion
- 2 tbspof freshly squeezed lime juice

Instructions

Add veggies to a bowl and mix. Drizzle lime juice and sprinkle using pepper and salt. Toss and enjoy your salad.

29 Fish Medley

(Ready in about 20 minutes | Serving 4 | Difficulty: Easy)

Per serving: Kcal 151, Fat: 3g, Net Carbs: 5.8, Protein: 24.4g

Ingredients

- 1 tsp sesame oil
- 1/2 cup scallions, thinly sliced
- 1/2 tsp fresh ginger, grated
- 1/2 tsp garlic, crushed
- 1 tsp red curry paste
- 2 whole star anise
- 1 tsp smoked paprika
- 2 ripe tomatoes, crushed
- Ground black pepper and sea salt
- 1 pound snapper, cut into bite-sized pieces

Instructions

Add oil to a pot and warm over moderate flame. Add ginger and scallions and cook for around 1 minute. Add the rest of the ingredients and reduce the flame. Simmer for around 15 minutes and enjoy.

30 Ham Wraps

(Ready in about 10 minutes | Serving 3 | Difficulty: Easy)

Per serving: Kcal 308, Fat: 19.9g, Net Carbs: 4.3g, Protein: 27.8g

Ingredients

- 1/2 cup dry white wine
- 1/2 cup water
- 1/2 tsp mixed peppercorns
- 1/2 tsp dry mustard powder
- 1/2 pound ahi tuna steak
- 6 slices of ham
- 1/2 Hass avocado, peeled, pitted and sliced
- 1 tbsp fresh lemon juice 6 lettuce leaves

Instructions

Add all the ingredients except lemon and avocado in a bowl and mix. Add to pan with tuna and simmer for around 5 minutes on each side. Slice the tuna after removing the liquid. Drizzle lemon over and add avocado. Roll wraps and place on a lettuce leaf.

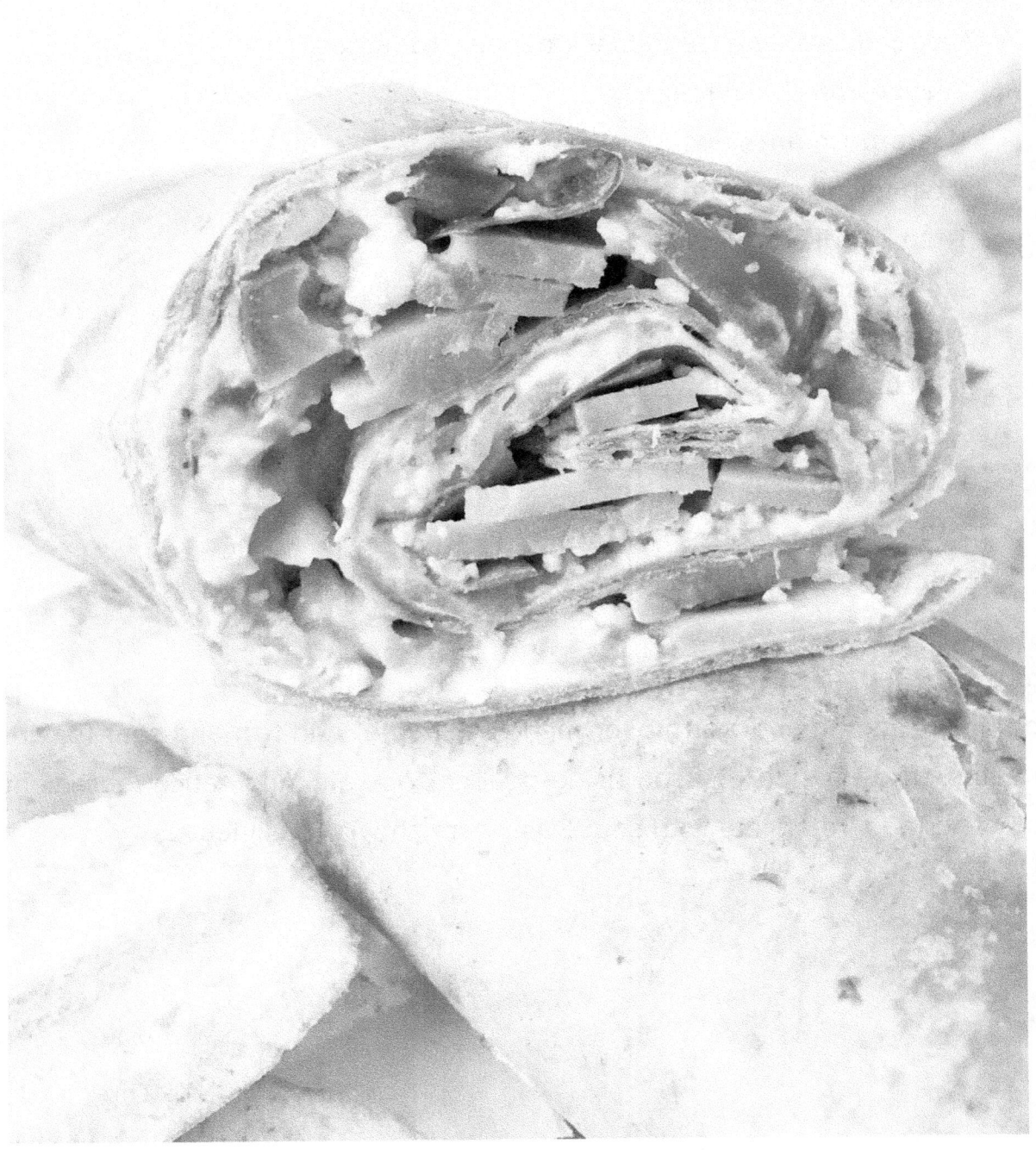

31 Alaskan Cod

(Ready in about 10 minutes | Serving 4 | Difficulty: Easy)

Per serving: Kcal 166, Fat: 8.2g, Net Carbs: 2.6g, Protein: 19.8g

Ingredients

- 1 tbsp coconut oil
- 4 Alaskan cod fillets
- Salt and freshly ground black pepper, to taste
- 6 leaves basil, chiffonade
- Mustard Cream Sauce:
- 1 tsp yellow mustard
- 1 tsp paprika
- 1/4 tsp ground bay leaf
- 3 tbsp cream cheese
- 1/2 cup Greek-style yogurt
- 1 garlic clove, minced
- 1 tsp lemon zest
- 1 tbsp fresh parsley, minced
- Sea salt and ground black pepper, to taste

Instructions

Add oil to the pan and warm over moderate flame. Add fish and sear for around 3 minutes on each side. Season using pepper and salt. Add sauce ingredients in a bowl and mix. Top fillets with sauce and garnish with basil leaves.

32 Paprika Omelet

(Ready in about 10 minutes | Serving 2 | Difficulty: Easy)

Per serving: Kcal 287, Fat: 22.6g, Net Carbs: 1.3g, Protein: 19.8g

Ingredients

- 2 tsp ghee, room temperature
- 4 eggs, whisked
- 4 tbsp goat cheese
- 1tsp paprika
- Sea salt and ground black pepper, to taste

Instructions

Add ghee to the pan and melt over moderate flame. Whisk eggs in a bowl and add to the pan. Cover the pan and reduce the flame to a low temperature. Cook for around 4 minutes. Add paprika and cheese and cook for 3 more minutes. Season using pepper and salt.

33 Boiled Eggs

(Ready in about 10 minutes | Serving 3 | Difficulty: Easy)

Per serving: Kcal 222, Fat: 17.6g, Net Carbs: 5.7g, Protein: 12.2

Ingredients

- 6 eggs
- 1/2 tsp kosher salt
- 1/2 tsp ground black pepper
- 1/2 tsp cayenne pepper
- 1/2 tsp dried dill weed
- 1 avocado, pitted and sliced
- 1tbsp lemon juice

Instructions

Add water to the pan and boil. Add eggs and cook for around 6 minutes on low heat. Peel eggs and cut them in half. Sprinkle with seasonings and drizzle lemon juice over avocado slices. Serve on the side with eggs.

34 Stuffed Peppers

(Ready in about 45 minutes | Serving 3 | Difficulty: Moderate)

Per serving: Kcal 194, Fat: 13.9g, Net Carbs: 3.5g, Protein: 13.3

Ingredients

- 3 bell peppers, halved, seeds removed
- 3 eggs, whisked
- 1 cup Mexican cheese blend
- 1 tsp chili powder
- 1 garlic clove, minced
- 1 tsp onion powder
- 1ripe tomato, pureed
- 1 tsp mustard powder

Instructions

Preheat the oven to 370 degrees F. Add oil to the pan and combine eggs, chili powder, cheese, onion powder and garlic in a bowl. Divide filling equally among bell peppers. Mix mustard powder and tomatoes and pour in pan. Bake for around 40 minutes, covered with foil

35 Kale Bake

(Ready in about 35 minutes | Serving 4 | Difficulty: Moderate)

Per serving: Kcal 384, Fat: 29.1g, Net Carbs: 5.9g, Protein: 25.1g

Ingredients

- Nonstick cooking spray
- 6 ounces kale, torn into pieces
- 4 eggs, whisked
- 1 cup Cheddar cheese, grated
- 1 cup Romano cheese
- 2 tbsp sour cream
- 1 garlic clove, minced
- Sea salt, to taste
- 1/2 tsp ground black pepper, or more to taste
- 1/2 tsp cayenne pepper

Instructions

Preheat the oven to 365 degrees F. Spray pan using cooking spray and mix everything in a bowl. Pour mixture into the prepared pan and bake for around 35 minutes.

36 Cheese Meatballs

(Ready in about 25 minutes | Serving 8 | Difficulty: Easy)

Per serving: Kcal 389, Fat: 31.3g, Net Carbs: 1.6g, Protein: 23.8

Ingredients

- 1/2 pound ground pork
- 1 pound ground turkey
- 1 garlic clove, minced
- 4tbsp pork rinds, crushed
- 2 tbsp shallots, chopped
- 4 ounces mozzarella string cheese, cubed
- 1 ripe tomato, pureed
- Salt and ground black pepper, to taste

Instructions

Combine all the ingredients in a bowl except cheese. Shape eatable balls out of this mixture. Add cheese cube in every ball and line a baking sheet with parchment paper. Place balls on a sheet and bake for around 25 minutes at around 350 degrees F.

37 Italian Crisps

(Ready in about 10 minutes | Serving 4 | Difficulty: Easy)

Per serving: Kcal 134, Fat: 11.1g, Net Carbs: 0.4g, Protein: 4.9g

Ingredients

- 1 cup sharp Cheddar cheese, grated
- 1/4 tsp ground black pepper
- 1/2tsp cayenne pepper
- 1 tsp Italian seasoning

Instructions

Preheat the oven to 400 degrees F and line parchment paper on a baking sheet. Mix everything in a bowl and pour onto a sheet in for of heaps of the size of a tbsp. Bake for around 8 minutes.

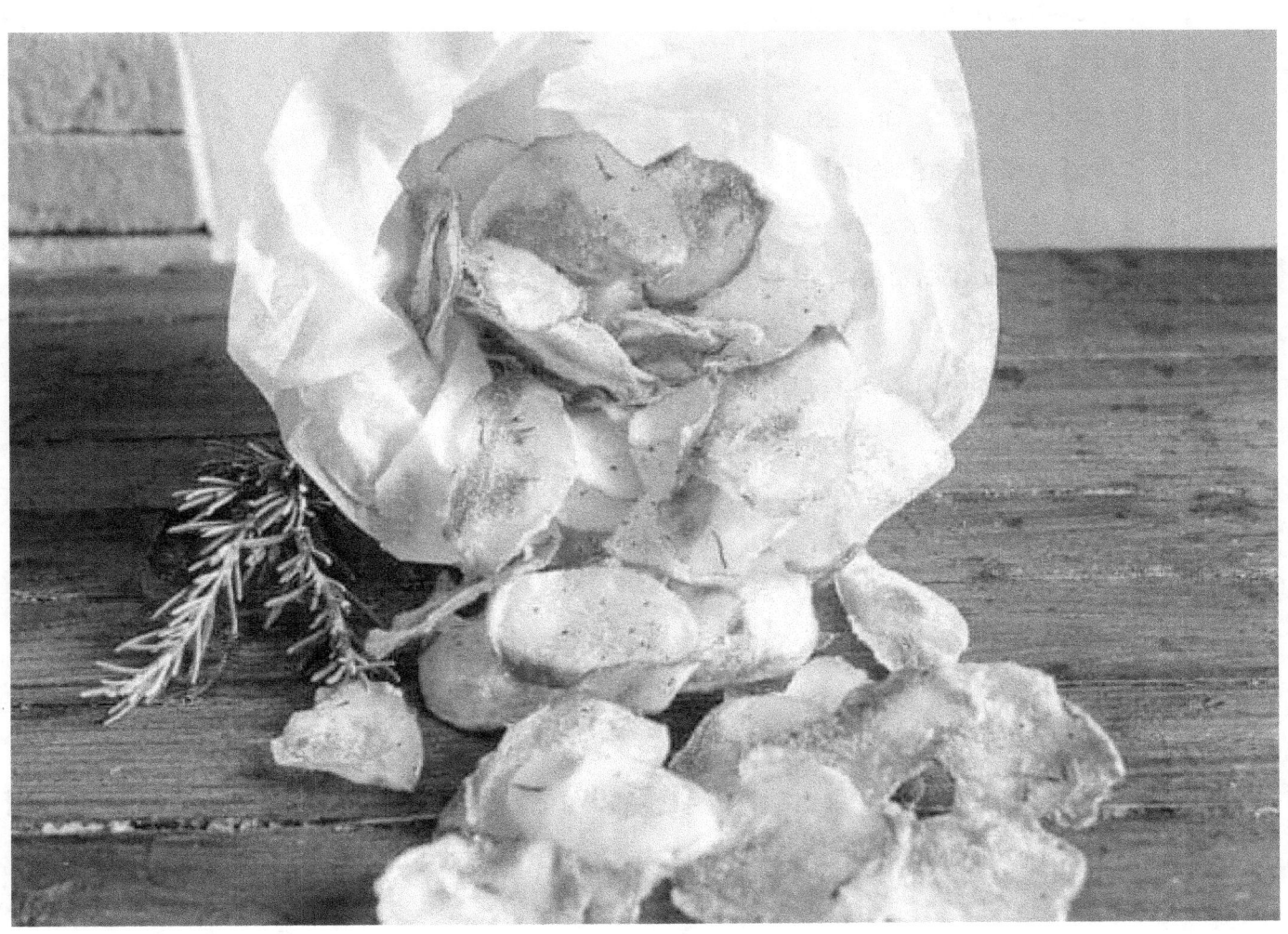

38 Spicy Meatballs

(Ready in about 15 minutes | Serving 3 | Difficulty: Easy)

Per serving: Kcal 458, Fat: 35.8g, Net Carbs: 4.3g, Protein: 28.2g

Ingredients

Sauce

- 3 ounces Asiago cheese, grated
- 1/4 cup mayonnaise
- 1 chili pepper, minced
- 1 tsp yellow mustard
- 1 tsp Italian parsley
- 1/2 tsp red pepper flakes, crushed
- 1/2 tsp sea salt
- 1/2 tsp ground black pepper

Meatballs

- 1/2 pound ground beef
- 1 egg
- 1 tbsp olive oil

Instructions

Add all the ingredients in the bowl except egg and beef and mix. Add egg and beef and combine thoroughly. Make meatballs out of the mixture. Warm oil in a pan placed on a moderate flame. Cook each side of meatballs for around 3 minutes.

39 Cheese Stuffed Mushrooms

(Ready in about 25 minutes | Serving 5 | Difficulty: Easy)

Per serving: Kcal 148, Fat: 8.4g, Net Carbs: 4.8g, Protein: 14.1g

Ingredients

- 4 ounces ground beef
- 2 ounces ground pork
- Kosher salt and ground black pepper, to taste
- 1/4 cup goat cheese, crumbled
- 2 tbsp Romano cheese, grated
- 2 tbsp shallot, minced
- 1 garlic clove, minced
- 1 tsp dried basil
- 1/2 tsp dried oregano
- 1/2 tsp dried rosemary
- 20 button mushrooms, stems removed

Instructions

Add everything except mushrooms in a bowl and mix. Stuff this mixture inside mushrooms. Preheat the oven to 370 degrees F. Bake these mushrooms in a pan for around 18 minutes.

40 Beef with Herbs

(Ready in about 50 minutes | Serving 4 | Difficulty: Moderate)

Per serving: Kcal 421, Fat: 35.7g, Net Carbs: 5.9g, Protein: 19.7g

Ingredients

- 1 tbsp olive oil
- 1 pound rib eye, cut into strips
- 2 tbsp rice wine
- 1/4cup beef bone broth
- Sea salt and ground black pepper, to taste
- 2 tbsp fresh parsley, finely chopped
- 2 tbsp fresh chives, finely chopped
- 2chipotle peppers in adobo sauce, chopped
- 1 garlic clove, crushed
- 2 small-sized ripe tomatoes, pureed
- 1 yellow onion, peeled and chopped
- 1/2 tsp dry mustard
- 1 tsp dried basil
- 1 tsp dried marjoram

Instructions

Warm oil in a pan placed on a moderate flame. Sear beef in pan for around 6 minutes. Reduce flame and add the rest of the ingredients and cook for around 40 minutes. Take the beef out and shred and enjoy.

41 Chinese Beef Skillet

(Ready in about 15 minutes | Serving 3 | Difficulty: Easy)

Per serving: Kcal 179, Fat: 10.4g, Net Carbs: 5.8g, Protein: 16.5g

Ingredients

- 1 tbsp sesame oil
- 1/2 pound ground chuck
- 1 shallot, minced
- 1 garlic clove, minced
- 1 (1/2-inch) piece ginger root, peeled and grated
- 1 bell pepper, seeded and sliced
- 4 ounces brown mushrooms, sliced
- 1 tsp tamari soy sauce
- 1 tbsp rice wine
- 2 whole star anise
- Himalayan salt and ground black pepper, to taste

Instructions

Warm oil in a pan over moderate flame and cook chuck until it changed its color. Then cook veggies in drippings inside the pan. Add rest of ingredients and beef to pan. Reduce flame and simmer for around 3 minutes.

42 Beef Stroganoff

(Ready in about 1 hour | Serving 4 | Difficulty: Hard)

Per serving: Kcal 303, Fat: 17.2g, Net Carbs: 5.6g, Protein: 32.4g

Ingredients

- 2 tbsp lard, room temperature
- 1 pound beef stew meat, cut across the grain into strips
- 1/2 yellow onion, peeled and chopped
- 2 garlic cloves, minced
- 4ounces fresh mushrooms, sliced
- 1/2 tsp salt
- 1 tsp smoked paprika
- 1/4tsp black pepper
- 1/2 tsp dried basil
- 1/4 cup red cooking wine
- 4 cups vegetable broth
- 1 fresh tomato, pureed
- 2 celery stalks, chopped
- 1/2 cup sour cream

Instructions

Place stockpot over moderate flame and melt the lard in it. Cook meat until it turns brown. Add garlic and onion and cook for around 1 minute. Add mushrooms, and until they turn tender, cook. Add rest of ingredients except sour cream and seasonings and simmer for around 50 minutes, covered. Add sour cream after turning the heat off and mix.

43 Chicken Zoodles

(Ready in about 19 minutes | Serving 4 | Difficulty: Easy)

Per serving: Kcal 411, Fat: 18.8g, Net Carbs: 11.7g, Protein: 45.7g

Ingredients

- 1/2 tsp of coconut butter
- 500 g of chicken fillets
- 1 medium onion diced
- 1 garlic minced
- Two zucchinis medium
- 400 g tomatoes crushed
- 100 g of raw cashews
- 7-10 chopped cherry tomatoes
- Salt, pepper, basil and oregano

Instructions

Warm pan over moderate flame. Cook butter and onions for around 1 minute. Make 2 cm pieces of chicken. Add garlic and chicken to the pan and sprinkle with seasonings. Cook for around 6 minutes. Spiralize zucchini in the meantime. Add tomatoes(crushed) and simmer for around 5 minutes. Roast cashews using another pan. Season with salt, paprika and turmeric. Add cherry tomatoes, zoodles and season using salt. Cook for another minute. Serve zoodles with fresh basil and cashews.

44 Creamy Tuscan Chicken

(Ready in about 25 minutes | Serving 6 | Difficulty: Easy)

Per serving: Kcal 368, Fat: 25g, Net Carbs: 7g, Protein: 30g

Ingredients

- 1 1/2 pounds of boneless skinless sliced chicken breasts
- 1 cup of heavy cream
- 1 cup chopped spinach
- 2 Tbsp of olive oil
- 1/2 cup of chicken broth
- 1 tsp of Italian seasoning
- 1 tsp of garlic powder
- 1/2 cup of parmesan cheese
- 1/2 cup of dried tomatoes

Instructions

Warm oil in a pan and cook each side of the chicken for around 5 minutes. Remove and place aside. Add everything except spinach and tomatoes to the pan and whisk over a moderate flame to form a thick mixture. Add tomatoes and spinach and simmer until spinach wilts. Add chicken and heat.

45 Turkey and peppers

(Ready in about 20 minutes | Serving 4 | Difficulty: Easy)

Per serving: Kcal 230, Fat: 8g, Net Carbs: 11g, Protein: 30g

Ingredients

- 1/2 large sliced sweet onion
- 1 pound cut into steaks turkey tenderloin
- 1 diced into strips yellow bell pepper
- 2 tbsp divided olive oil extra-virgin
- 1 diced into strips red bell pepper
- 1 tsp divided salt
- 1/2tsp of Italian seasoning
- 2 tsp of red wine vinegar
- 1/4tsp of ground black pepper
- 1 14-ounce can of crushed tomatoes

Instructions

Sprinkle turkey with half tsp salt. Warm 1 tbsp oil in a pan and cook half of the turkey for around 3 minutes. Transfer to a plate and add remaining oil to the pan. Repeat with the rest of the turkey. Add veggies and half tsp salt to the pan and cook for around 7 minutes. Sprinkle with seasoning plus pepper and cook on a moderate flame for around 30 seconds. Add vinegar and cook for another 20 seconds. Add turkey to the pan and simmer for around 2 minutes. Top with basil and parsley.

46 Butter Chicken

(Ready in about 30 minutes | Serving 6 | Difficulty: Easy)

Per serving: Kcal 293, Fat: 17g, Net Carbs: 9g, Protein: 29g

Ingredients

- 1.5 lbs cubed chicken breast
- 4 oz plain Greek yogurt whole milk
- 3 tsp grated fresh ginger
- 2 tbsp of garam masala
- 3 tsp garlic minced
- 1 tbsp of coconut oil

Sauce

- 2 tbsp of butter
- 2 tsp grated fresh ginger
- 1/2 cup of heavy cream
- 2 tsp garlic minced
- 14.5 oz can tomatoes crushed
- 1 onion
- 1 tbsp coriander ground
- 2 tsp of cumin
- 1/2tbsp of garam masala
- 1 tsp of chili powder
- Salt

Instructions

Dice chicken into pieces of 2 inch and mix with garam masala, 1 tsp each of garlic and ginger in a bowl. Add yogurt and mix. Place in the fridge for around 30 minutes. Add tomatoes, garlic, ginger, spices and onion in a blender and blend to make a smooth mixture. Place aside. Warm 1 tbsp oil in a pan and add marinade and chicken. Cook each side for around 4 minutes. Add sauce and cook for 6 more minutes. Add ghee and heavy cream and cook for an additional minute. Top using cilantro.

47 Asparagus Chicken

(Ready in about 30 minutes | Serving 3 | Difficulty: Easy)

Per serving: Kcal 572, Fat: 31g, Net Carbs: 10g, Protein: 62g

Ingredients

- 3 Breasts Chicken
- 12 Stalks removed Asparagus
- 1 cup of mozzarella shredded
- 1 tsp of Garlic paste
- 1/2 cup of Cream Cheese
- 1 tsp of Olive Oil
- 1 tbsp of Butter
- 3/4 cup of Marinara Sauce
- Pepper and salt

Instructions

Slice chicken without cutting from the center. Cut stalks from asparagus. Rub garlic paste, salt and pepper over chicken and spread with cream cheese. Place 4 asparagus stalks in the center and fold the breasts. Preheat the oven to 400 degrees F and cook each side for around 7 minutes. Top with marinara sauce and mozzarella. Broil for around 5 minutes.

48 Chicken Chili

(Ready in about 30 minutes | Serving 6 | Difficulty: Easy)

Per serving: Kcal 201, Fat: 11g, Net Carbs: 7g, Protein: 18g

Ingredients

- 4 shredded chicken breasts
- 2 cups of Chicken broth
- 1 tbsp of Butter
- 1/2 chopped onion
- 10 oz canned diced tomatoes, undrained
- 4 oz of Cream cheese
- 2 oz of tomato paste
- 1 tbsp of Cumin
- 1 tbsp of Chili powder
- 1/2 tbsp of Garlic powder
- Pepper and salt

Instructions

Boil chicken in broth for around 12 minutes. Take out and shred. Melt butter in a pot over moderate flame and cook the onion for around 2 minutes. Add chicken and rest of the ingredients except cream cheese in pot and stir. Boil and reduce the flame to simmer for around 10 minutes. Cut cream into chunks of 1 inch. Add to pot and stir until mixed. Season using pepper and salt.

49 Taco Avocados

(Ready in about 20 minutes | Serving 6 | Difficulty: Easy)

Per serving: Kcal 401, Fat: 28g, Net Carbs: 5g, Protein: 26g

Ingredients

- 1 pound beef ground
- 1/2 tsp of Salt
- 1 tbsp of Chili Powder
- 1/2 tsp of Dried Oregano
- 3/4 tsp of Cumin
- 1/4 tsp of Garlic Powder
- 4 ounces of tomato sauce
- 1/4 tsp of Onion Powder
- 3 halved avocados
- 1 cup shredded cheddar cheese
- 1/4 cup sliced cherry tomatoes
- 1/4 cup shredded lettuce

Instructions

Add beef to a pan and cook until it turns brown. Remove grease and mix tomato sauce and seasonings. Cook for around 4 minutes and take the pit out of avocados. Load taco meat in crater and top with tomatoes, cheese, sour cream, cilantro and lettuce.

50 Broccoli Beef Bowls

(Ready in about 30 minutes | Serving 4 | Difficulty: Easy)

Per serving: Kcal 388, Fat: 29g, Net Carbs: 14g, Protein: 30g

Ingredients

Beef

- 1 pound grass-fed beef ground
- 1 tsp of granulated garlic
- 1 tsp of fine salt
- 1 tbsp of cooking fat
- 1 tbsp of coconut aminos

Broccoli

- 4 diced into florets broccoli crowns
- 1/2 tsp of fine salt
- 1 tbsp of avocado oil

Sunshine Sauce

- 1 tbsp of cooking fat
- 1/2 of fine salt
- 2 tbsp seed sunflower butter
- 2 tsp of coconut aminos
- 1 tsp of ground ginger
- one lemon, juiced
- 1 minced green onion
- 1/4 cup of bone broth

To assemble

- 4 cups of baby spinach

Instructions

Preheat oven to around 400 degrees F. Mix salt and fat with broccoli on pan and massage fat into florets. Cook for around 20 minutes. Crumble beef in a pan and add garlic and salt. Stir and add coconut aminos and turn flame to high. Cook until beef turns crispy and brown. Place a pot on moderate flame and melt fat in it. Add seed butter and sunflower and stir to make a smooth mixture. Add rest of ingredients except lemon juice and stir. Take off the heat and mix lemon juice. Add baby spinach to 4 bowls and divide beef equally. Add broccoli florets and top with sauce.

51 Cauliflower-Bacon Cheese Mash

(Ready in about 15 minutes | Serving 4 | Difficulty: Easy)

Per serving: Kcal 399, Fat: 32.2g, Sodium 877.8mg, Protein: 18.8g

Ingredients

- 1 cauliflower, large head, diced into florets
- ½ lb. bacon, diced
- 1 cup of Parmesan cheese, shredded
- 2 tbsp. medium-chain triglyceride oil
- 4 tbsp. unsalted butter
- Sea salt to taste
- ½ tbsp. apple cider vinegar

Instruction

- Cook the bacon in a big skillet over the medium-high flame, sometimes flipping, for five to ten minutes or evenly browned. Reserve the grease in the skillet and drain on the paper towels.
- In a pressure cooker, place the cauliflower in a metal or silicone steamer basket. Fill the container with 1 cup of water. Cover the lid and lock it. Set the timer for four minutes and select the Steam function. Allow for a ten to a fifteen-minute build-up of pressure.
- Pressure can be released slowly and cautiously using the quick-release system according to the manufacturer's directions, which should take around five minutes. Remove the lid by unlocking it.
- Drain the cauliflower and put it in a big mixing bowl. Combine the Parmesan cheese, butter, MCT oil, vinegar, and salt in a mixing bowl. Using an immersion blender, blend until absolutely smooth. Add the sliced bacon and mix properly. Add one or two teaspoons of the bacon grease that has been put aside.

52 Spaghetti Squash With Blue Cheese And Bacon

(Ready in about 15 minutes | Serving 2 | Difficulty: Easy)
Per serving: Kcal 339, Fat: 24.3g, Sodium 691.2mg, Protein: 13.5g

Ingredients
- 1 tbsp. olive oil
- 1 spaghetti squash, small
- Ground black pepper and salt according to taste
- 2 tbsp. crumbled blue cheese
- 1 (4 oz.) sliced package mushrooms
- 4 slices bacon, diced into 1/2-inch pieces
- 1 clove minced garlic
- ¼ cup of sour cream
- 2 cup of baby spinach

Instruction
- Preheat oven to 400 degrees Fahrenheit. Aluminum foil can be used to line a baking sheet.
- Using a sharp knife, cut the stem from the end of the spaghetti squash. Squash can be cut in half lengthwise, and the seeds scraped off. Brush with olive oil and season with salt and pepper.
- Bake for forty-five minutes in a preheated oven till tender. Remove the fried flesh to a bowl and put it aside. Return the shells of the spaghetti squash to the baking sheet.
- Cook the bacon in a big skillet over medium-high flame, sometimes flipping, for five to six minutes, or till evenly browned. On paper towels, drain the bacon slices.
- Cook for four to five minutes with the garlic and mushrooms in the skillet. In a large mixing bowl, combine the spinach and cooked bacon. Stir for two to three minutes or till spinach is wilted. Toss the mushroom

mixture into the squash bowl. Combine the salt, pepper, and sour cream in a mixing bowl. Stir until all of the fillings are distributed.
- Fill the squash shells with the filling. On each half, sprinkle 1 tbsp. blue cheese. Return to oven and bake for another four to five minutes, or till the cheese has melted and the squash has cooked through.

53 Ranch Cauliflower Crackers

(Ready in about 20 minutes | Serving 18 | Difficulty: Easy)
Per serving: Kcal 29, Fat: 1.5g, Sodium 103.5mg, Protein: 2.5g

Ingredients
- Cheesecloth
- 1 (12 oz.) frozen riced cauliflower
- 1 cup of Parmesan cheese, shredded
- 1 egg
- ⅛ tsp. cayenne pepper, or according to taste
- 1 tbsp. salad dressing mix, dry ranch

Instructions
- In a microwave-safe bowl, put the riced cauliflower. Microwave for three to four minutes, covered. Allow it to cool for fifteen minutes in a strainer lined with cheesecloth. Squeeze the moisture out of the riced cauliflower after it has cooled.
- Preheat oven to 425 degrees Fahrenheit. Using parchment paper, line the baking dish.
- In a mixing bowl, combine the egg, riced cauliflower, cayenne pepper, and ranch blend. Stir in the Parmesan cheese till it is fully incorporated.
- With a tiny cookie scoop, transfer the mixture onto a prepared cookie sheet and flatten it to around 1/16-inch thickness with a tiny hand-rolling pin, cup, or your hand. The crispier your cracker is, the thinner the dough will be.
- Bake for ten minutes in a preheated oven, then flip and bake for another ten minutes. Allow cooling on a wire shelf.

54 Easy Cauliflower Casserole

(Ready in about 10 minutes | Serving 2 | Difficulty: Easy)

Per serving: Kcal 469, Fat: 40.9g, Sodium 494.1mg, Protein: 18.1g

Ingredients
- 1 cup of Cheddar cheese, shredded
- ½ head cauliflower florets
- 1 pinch freshly ground black pepper and salt or according to taste
- ½ cup of heavy cream

Instruction
- Preheat oven to 400 degrees Fahrenheit.
- Cook the cauliflower in a big pot of lightly salted water until soft yet firm to the bite, approximately ten minutes. Drain.
- In a big mixing bowl, combine the cream, Cheddar cheese, pepper, and salt. Cover cauliflower with the cheese mixture in a casserole dish.
- Bake for twenty-five minutes in a preheated oven till the cheese is golden brown and bubbly.

55 White Chicken Chili

(Ready in about 20 minutes | Serving 8 | Difficulty: Easy)
Per serving: Kcal 591, Fat: 49.6g, Sodium 795mg, Protein: 31.8g

Ingredients

- 1 stick divide butter
- 1 tbsp. oil, or as required
- 2 lb. Boneless, skinless, chicken breasts
- Ground black pepper and salt according to taste
- 1 ½ tsp. chili powder
- ¾ cup of chicken broth
- 4 oz. cream cheese
- 2 cup of heavy whipping cream
- 1 ½ tbsp. onion powder
- 1 tsp. hot sauce
- 2 tsp. cumin
- 2 (4 oz.) cans green chilies, chopped
- 1 ½ cup of Monterey Jack cheese, grated

Instruction

- Add oil and two tbsp. Butter to a big skillet and cook over medium-high flame.
- Season the chicken with salt, black pepper, and chili powder in the meantime. Cook the chicken in skillet for five minutes, on the one hand, resisting the temptation to turn it too soon. Cook, sometimes flipping to avoid burning, until the insides are no longer pink and the juices run free, approximately ten to fifteen minutes, relying on thickness. Transfer the chicken to the plate to cool for ten minutes or before it is ready to handle. Set aside chicken that has been shredded with your fingertips.

- In a big, heavy pot, combine the remaining 6 tbsp. Butter, heavy cream, chicken broth, cream cheese, cumin, hot sauce, and onion powder. Season with the black pepper and salt, then reduce to low heat and cook for five minutes, or until the butter and cream cheese have melted.
- To the chili in a pot, add shredded chicken, Monterey Jack cheese, and green chiles. Reduce the heat to low and simmer for twenty minutes, stirring occasionally.

Conclusion

A keto diet may be a healthier option for certain people, although the amount of fat, carbohydrates, and protein prescribed varies from person to person. If you have diabetes, talk to the doctor before starting the diet because it would almost certainly need prescription changes and stronger blood sugar regulation. Are you taking drugs for high blood pressure? Before starting a keto diet again, talk to the doctor. If you're breastfeeding, you shouldn't follow a ketogenic diet. Be mindful that limiting carbs will render you irritable, hungry, and sleepy, among other things. However, this may be a one-time occurrence. Keep in mind that you can eat a balanced diet in order to obtain all of the vitamins and minerals you need. A sufficient amount of fiber is also needed. When the body begins to derive energy from accumulated fat rather than glucose, it is said to be in ketosis. Several trials have shown the powerful weight-loss benefits of a low-carb, or keto, diet. This diet, on the other hand, can be difficult to stick to and can exacerbate health issues in individuals who have certain disorders, such as diabetes type 1. The keto diet is suitable for the majority of citizens. Nonetheless, all major dietary modifications should be discussed with a dietitian or doctor. This is essentially the case with people who have inherent conditions. The keto diet may be an effective therapy for people with drug-resistant epilepsy. Though the diet may be beneficial to people of any age, teenagers, people over 50, and babies can profit the most because they can easily stick to it. Modified keto diets, such as the revised Atkins diet or the low-glycemic index diet, are safer for adolescents and adults. A health care worker should keep a careful eye on someone who is taking a keto diet as a treatment. A doctor and dietitian will maintain track of a person's progress, administer drugs, and test for side effects. The body absorbs fat and protein differently than it does carbohydrates. Carbohydrates have a high insulin reaction. The protein sensitivity to insulin is mild, and the quick insulin response is negligible. Insulin is a fat-producing and fat-conserving enzyme. If you wish to lose weight, consume as many eggs, chickens, fish, and birds as you want, satiate yourself with the fat, and then eat every vegetable that grows on the ground. Butter and coconut oil can be used instead of processed synthetic seed oils. You may be either a sugar or a fat burner, but not both.

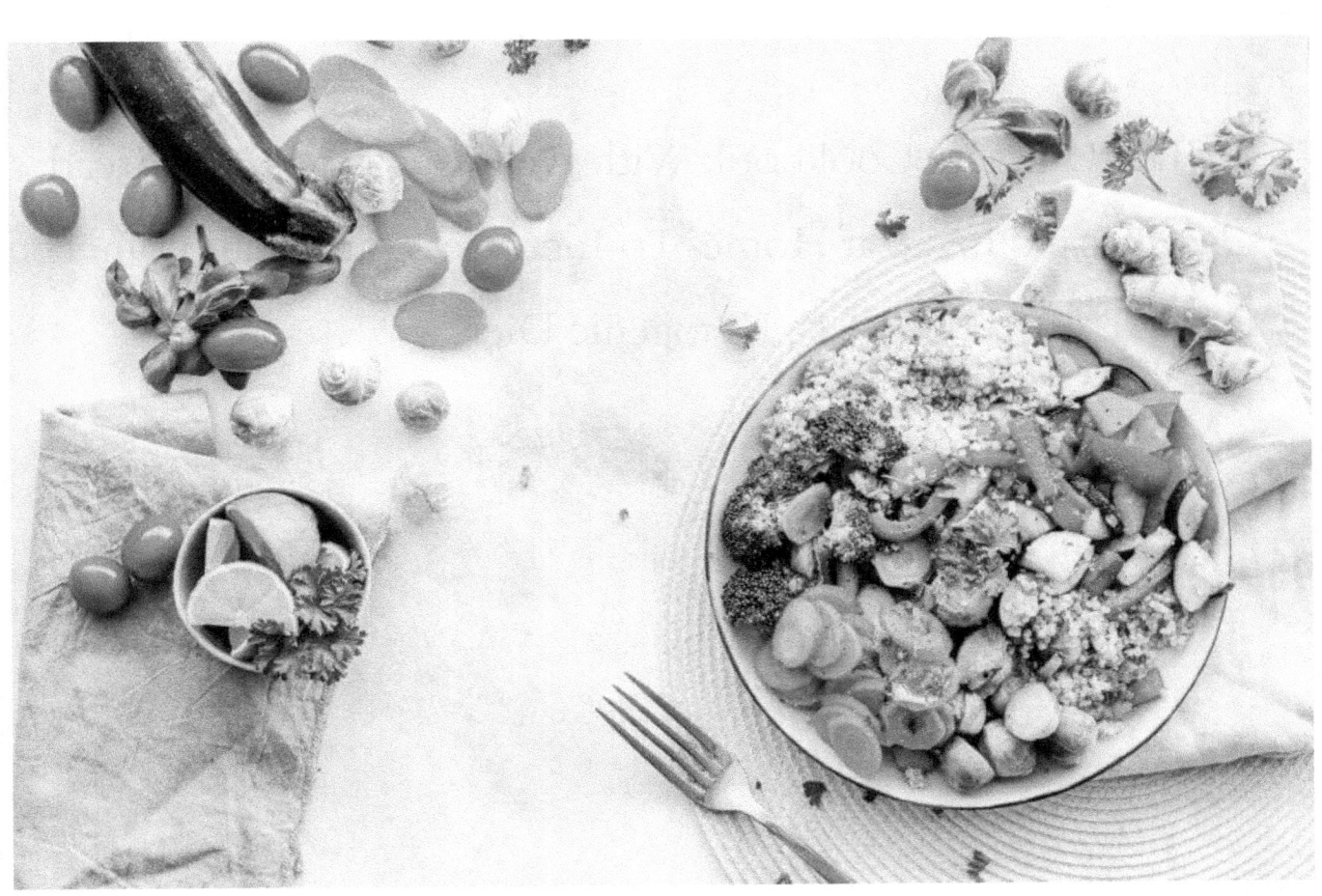

Essential Keto Bread

The Ultimate Cookbook With Delicious Low Carb Bread Recipes To make at Home, To Increase Your Health On The Ketogenic Diet

By

Sofia Wilson

Introduction

Ketogenic refers to a low-carbohydrate diet. The aim is to eat more calories from fat and protein while eating fewer calories from carbohydrates. The carbohydrates that are easiest to digest, such as starch, pastries, soda, and white bread, are the first to go. When you consume fewer than 50 g of carbohydrates a day, your body easily runs out of energy. This normally takes three or four days. Then you'll begin to break down fat and protein for energy, potentially resulting in weight loss. Ketosis is the term for this state. It's crucial to remember that the ketogenic diet is a short-term diet designed to help you lose weight rather than change your lifestyle. A ketogenic diet is more often used to reduce weight, although it may also be used to treat medical problems such as epilepsy. It can even benefit those suffering from heart failure, some brain disorders, and even acne, although further study is required. Since the keto diet contains too much fat, adherents must ingest fat at every meal time. In a normal 2K-calorie diet, that would seem like 165 g of fat, 40 g of carbohydrates, and 75 g of protein. The exact ratio, on the other hand, is determined by your basic requirements. Nuts (walnuts, almonds), avocados, seeds, olive oil and tofu are among the healthier unsaturated fats allowed on the keto diet. However, oils (coconut, palm), butter, lard, and peanut butter all contain high amounts of saturated fats. Protein is an essential aspect of the keto diet, although it is also difficult to discern between protein items that are lean and protein products rich in fat(saturated), such as beef, bacon, and pork. What for fruits and vegetables? While fruits are generally rich in carbohydrates, unique fruits may be obtained in limited quantities (generally berries) Leafy greens (like kale, chard, Swiss chard, and spinach), broccoli, cauliflower, asparagus, tomatoes, brussels sprouts, bell peppers, garlic, cucumbers, mushrooms, summer squashes, as well as celery are also rich in carbohydrates. One cup of sliced broccoli includes about six carbohydrates. At the same time, there are several possible keto hazards, such as liver deficiency, liver complications, constipation, kidney disorders, and so on. As a result, we can also keep our Keto diet portions in check.

Understanding The Ketogenic Diet

This chapter delves into the Ketogenic diet in depth. The chapter further discusses which foods to consume on the Keto diet and which foods to stop while on this diet. The Keto diet is often explained in-depth, including how it functions and what health advantages it provides.

The ketogenic diet (or keto diet) is a high-fat, low-carbohydrate diet with various health benefits. Evidently, more than 20 studies suggest that this form of diet will help you lose weight and boost your wellbeing. Diabetes patients, epilepsy patients, patients suffering from Alzheimer's disease, as well as cancer can all benefit from ketogenic diets.

1.1 What is Keto?

The ketogenic diet is a very low carbohydrate, high-fat diet that has a lot in common with the Atkins diet and other low-carb diets. It necessitates a significant reduction of carbohydrate consumption and a replacement with fat. This reduction of carbohydrates puts the body into a metabolic condition known as ketosis. As this occurs, the body's energy production of fat-burning skyrockets. In addition, it converts fat into ketones in the liver, which will supply energy to the brain. Ketogenic diets can result in substantial reductions in insulin as well as blood sugar levels. This, along with the increased ketones, has numerous health benefits.

Ketogenic Diets Come in Many Forms

There are a few variations of the ketogenic diet, including:

The traditional ketogenic diet consists of a diet that is low in carbs, mild in protein, and strong in fats. It usually has a 75 percent fat content, a 5% carbohydrate content, and a 20% protein content.

The cyclic ketogenic diet entails high-carb reefed cycles, such as five ketogenic days accompanied by two days of high carbohydrate use.

A ketogenic diet with particular goals: The diet requires carbs to be inserted in between exercises.

Protein-rich ketogenic diet: This is comparable to a normal keto diet, but it contains extra protein. Usually, the ratio is 60 percent fat, 5% sugars, and 35 percent protein.

However, only normal and protein-rich ketogenic diets have been extensively studied. More complex keto diets, such as targeted or cyclic keto, are mainly utilized by bodybuilders and athletes.

Ketogenic Diet Health Benefits

In fact, the keto diet first gained popularity as a means of treating neurological conditions, such as epilepsy. Following that, research has shown that diet can help with a broad variety of health issues:

Heart disease: The keto diet has been found to decrease risk factors such as body fat, blood sugar, HDL cholesterol and blood pressure.

Alzheimer's disease: The ketogenic diet can ease Alzheimer's symptoms while still delaying the disease's progression.

Epilepsy: Research has demonstrated that a ketogenic diet can significantly reduce seizures in children with epileptic seizures.

Cancer: The diet is actually being used to control a number of diseases and to delay tumor development.

Acne: Lower insulin levels, as well as less sugar or fried food diets, will aid acne recovery.

Parkinson's disease: According to one report, diet can help relieve the effects of Parkinson's disease.

Brain injuries: One study found that the diet would also increase concussions and improve recovery after a brain injury.

Polycystic ovary syndrome: A ketogenic diet may help lower insulin levels and can be helpful in the treatment of polycystic ovary syndrome.

What foods can you consume on a ketogenic diet?

The majority of your meals will revolve around the following foods:
- Salmon, mackerel and tuna are representations of fatty fish.
- Look for pastured eggs, whole eggs, or omega-3 eggs.
- Seek for grass-fed butter plus cream wherever possible.
- Red meat, ham, sausage, turkey, bacon, chicken and steak are all examples of meat.
- Non-processed cheese (goat, cheddar, mozzarella, blue, or cream).
- Flax seeds, walnuts, almonds, pumpkin seeds, chia seeds and other nuts and beans
- Avocado oil, olive oil and coconut oil are the other safe oils.
- Salt, spices and pepper, as well as a variety of herbs, may be used as condiments.
- Avocados: entire avocados or guacamole made freshly.
- Low-carb vegetables including greens, tomatoes, onions, peppers and other related veggies.

Foods to avoid on a ketogenic diet include:

Carbohydrate-rich diets can be avoided as much as possible.

The following is a selection of items that must be eliminated or reduced on a ketogenic diet:
- Sugary drink, ice cream, soda, smoothies, cake, candy and other sugary items
- Wheat, pasta, cereals, rice, and other wheat-based products are examples of starches or grains.
- Sweet potatoes, parsnips, parsnips, potatoes, carrots and other tubers & root vegetables
- Reduced-calorie or low-fat foods are extremely processed and abundant in carbohydrates.
- Fruit: All fruits, with the exception of tiny bits of berries like strawberries.
- Chickpeas, lentils, peas, kidney beans, and other legumes or beans

- Some sauces/condiments: They are also high in unhealthy fat and sugar.
- Unhealthy fats: Limit the intake to mayonnaise, processed vegetable oils, and other processed fats.
- Alcohol: Because of their carb content, certain alcoholic beverages will shake you out of ketosis.
- Dietary ingredients that are sugar-free: Alcohols, which are often rich in sugar, may influence ketone levels in certain situations. These objects seem to have passed through a lot of refining as well.

1.2 What is the Keto diet, and how does it work?

The "ketogenic" keto diet consists of consuming a moderate level of protein, a heavy amount of fat, and relatively little carbohydrates; also, the fruit is forbidden. As for every diet fad, the advantages to adherents include improved vitality, weight reduction, and mental clarity. Is the ketogenic diet, though, what it's cracked up to be?

Dietitians and nutritionists are quiet on the topic. Low-carb diets like keto appear to assist with weight loss in the short term, but they are no more successful than any other self-help or conventional diet. They still don't seem to be enhancing athletic results.

The ketogenic diet was created to treat epilepsy instead of losing weight. In the 1920s, physicians found that holding people on low-carb diets induced their bodies to use fat as the predominant fuel source rather than glucose. When only fat is available for the body to combust or burn, the body converts fats to fatty acids, which are then converted to ketones, which can be used and taken up to power the body's cells.

Currently, feeding the body exclusively ketones prevents epilepsy for unclear causes. However, with the advent of anti-seizure medicines, few patients with epilepsy rely on ketogenic diets anymore, while certain people who may not respond to medications may benefit. Low carb diets like the Atkins diet, which gained popularity in the early 2000s, also spawned keto diets for weight loss. In comparison, all groups of meatier-meal diets restrict carbohydrates. This diet does not have a set structure, although most routines provide for fewer than fifty grams of carbs per day.

A keto diet causes the body to enter a state known as ketosis, in which the body's cells become completely reliant on ketones for nutrition. It's not exactly clear that this leads to weight loss, but ketosis decreases appetite and can affect hunger-controlling hormones, including insulin. As a consequence, proteins and fats can keep humans fuller longer than sugars, resulting in lower net calorie intake.

In one head-to-head comparison, researchers looked at 48 separate diet trials in which subjects were randomly allocated to one of the well-known diets. Low-carb diets like South Beach, Atkins, and Zone, as well as low-fat diets like Ornish diets and portion restriction diets like Weight Watchers and Jenny Craig, were among the options.

Every diet resulted in greater weight loss than almost no diet after six months, according to the results. Low-carb and low-fat dieters lost almost equal amounts of weight as compared to non-dieters, with low-carb dieters losing 19 pounds on average versus low-fat dieters dropping 17.6 pounds (7.99 kilograms). At 12 months, both diet styles displayed symptoms of dropping off, with low-fat and low-carb dieters being 16 pounds (7.27 kg) smaller on average than non-dieters.

There were few differences in weight reduction within the diets of designated people. This is in line with the practice of recommending every diet that an individual practice in order to lose weight.

Another study of well-known diets discovered the Atkins diet, which results in greater weight loss than merely teaching people about portion control. Nevertheless, several of the scientific researched about this low-carb diet featured licensed dietitians assisting respondents in making food decisions, rather than the self-directed approach used by most people. This has been seen in other diet studies, according to the researchers, and the tests' results seem to be more positive in the real world than the weight loss.

Finally, a simple comparison between low-carb versus low-fat dieting revealed that there was a statistically significant difference in the amount of weight lost over a year. Low-carbohydrate dieters dropped an average of 13 pounds (6 kg), compared to 11.7 pounds for low-fat dieters (5.3 kg).

Ketogenic diets may help us lose weight, but they are no more successful than other diet methods. Since carbohydrate reserves in the body comprise water molecules, the bulk of the weight lost during the early stages of a ketogenic diet is water weight. This gives the scale an exciting amount at first, but weight reduction slows down with time.

What are the keto effects, and how can they help?

The advantages of a keto diet are close to that of other high-fat, low-carb diets, but it tends to be more successful than centrist low-carb diets. Keto is a low-carb, high-fat diet that maximizes health benefits. However, it will slightly raise the likelihood of complications.

Aid in weight loss

Weight reduction can be improved by converting the body into a fat-burning device. Insulin levels – the hormone that retains fat – are falling rapidly, suggesting that fat burning has risen dramatically. This seems to make it much easier to lose bodyweight without going hungry.

More than thirty high-quality observational studies show that low-carb and keto diets are more effective than other diets at losing weight.

Reverse type 2 diabetes by regulating blood sugar

A ketogenic diet has been shown in research to be successful in the treatment of type 2 diabetes, with total disease reversal occurring in certain instances. It makes perfect sense since keto removes the need for therapy, lowers blood sugar levels, and eliminates the potential negative consequences of high insulin levels.

Since a keto diet will reverse type 2 diabetes, it is likely to be helpful in preventing and reversing pre-diabetes. Keep in mind that "reversal" in this context refers to changing the disease, improving glucose tolerance, and reducing the need for care. It may be so drastically altered that after therapy, blood pressure returns to normal with time. In this context, reversal refers to progressing or deteriorating in the reverse direction of the condition. Changes in your lifestyle, on the other side, just succeed if you bring them into effect. If a person returns to the way of life he or she has before diabetes type 2 appeared and advanced, it is possible that success would return with time.

Improve your mental and physical performance:
Some people use ketogenic diets to boost their mental performance. It's also normal for people to feel more energized while they're in ketosis.
They don't need nutritional carbs for the brain on keto. It runs on ketones 24 hours a day, seven days a week, with a small amount of glucose synthesized in the liver. Carbohydrates are not necessary for the diet. As a result, ketosis leads to a steady flow of food (ketones) to the brain, avoiding significant blood sugar spikes. This will also assist with improved focus and attention, as well as clearing brain fog and improving mental awareness.

Epilepsy Treatment

The keto diet has been used to manage epilepsy since the 19th and 20th centuries and has proved to be effective. It has historically been used mainly for adolescents, although in recent years, it has also proved to be useful to adults. Or, used in conjunction with a keto diet, certain people with epilepsy might be able to take less to no anti-epileptic drugs while being seizure-free. This may help to reduce the drug's adverse effects while still improving cognitive capacity.

Keto Bread Recipes

1 Empanadas

(Ready in about 35 minutes | Serving 4 | Difficulty: Moderate)

Per serving: Kcal 554, Fat: 48g, Net Carbs: 7g, Protein: 19g

Ingredients

- 11/4 cups of almond flour
- 1/2 tsp of cream of tartar
- 1 tsp of whipping cream
- 1 tsp of baking powder
- 1 tsp of xanthan gum
- 2 tbsp of butter
- 2 eggs
- 2 tbsp of ricotta cheese

Instructions

Mix everything except half of the eggs in a bowl. Knead using the mixer's hook attachment until a ball of dough is formed. Use plastic film to wrap it and place it in the fridge for around an hour. Make squared of parchment paper. Take the dough out and dice it into pieces and make a ball out of each piece. Press every ball between 2 pieces of paper to form a flat disk. Peel the paper on the top side and use it for the rest of the balls. Split the rest of the egg into white and yolk. Whisk heavy cream and yolk. Brush balls with it and place them on a baking tray. Bake for around 20 minutes at 300 degrees F.

2 Keto bagels

(Ready in about 25 minutes | Serving 4 | Difficulty: Easy)

Per serving: Kcal 477, Fat: 39g, Net Carbs: 4g, Protein: 23g

Ingredients

Bagels

- 1 egg
- 7 oz. of mozzarella cheese
- 1 1/2 cups of almond flour
- 1 oz. of cream cheese
- 2 tsp of baking powder

Topping

- 1 tsp of sesame seeds
- 2 tsp of flaxseed
- 1/2 tsp of sea salt
- 1 egg
- 1/4 tsp of poppy seeds

Instructions

Preheat oven to around 430 degrees F. Line parchment paper in the baking tray. Microwave cream cheese and mozzarella in a bowl for around 1 minute. Whisk baking powder and flour in another bowl. Add egg with this mixture into cheese. Whisk to form a dough. Divide dough into 4 parts and make bun shapes. Place on a tray and form a hole in the center using the thumb. Place seasoning and seeds in a bowl and stir. Beat one more egg in a bowl and brush bagel with it. Sprinkle seasoning and bake for around 15 minutes.

3 Hot dog buns

(Ready in about 1 hour | Serving 10 | Difficulty: Hard)

Per serving: Kcal 311, Fat: 8g, Net Carbs: 1g, Protein: 4g

Ingredients

- 1 1/4 cups of almond flour
- 2 tsp of baking powder
- 1/3 cup of psyllium husk ground
- 1 tsp of sea salt
- 1 1/4 cups of boiling water
- 2 tsp of cider vinegar
- 3 eggs, only whites

Instructions

Preheat oven to around 350 degrees F. Mix dry ingredients using a bowl. Boil water and add egg whites and vinegar in a bowl and mix for around 30 seconds using a hand mixer. Make 10 pieces out of dough and roll into the shape of hot dog buns. Place in a tray and bake for around 50 minutes.

4 Cornbread

(Ready in about 25 minutes | Serving 8 | Difficulty: Easy)

Per serving: Kcal 237, Fat: 23g, Net Carbs: 1g, Protein: 7g

Ingredients

- 1/4 cup of coconut flour
- 1/3 cup of whey protein
- 1/3 cup of oat fiber
- 11/2 tsp of baking powder
- 4 oz. melted butter
- 1/4 tsp of salt
- 1/3 cup of bacon fat
- 4 eggs
- 1/4 cup of water
- 1/4 tsp corn of extract

Instructions

Preheat oven to around 350 degrees F. Oil a pan and warm in the oven. Mix dry ingredients using a bowl and add the rest of the ingredients except corn extract. Beat using a hand mixer and add corn extract. Pour mixture into the pan and bake for around 20 minutes.

5 Quick style bread

(Ready in about 15 minutes | Serving 4 | Difficulty: Easy)

Per serving: Kcal 303, Fat: 26g, Net Carbs: 5g, Protein: 10g

Ingredients

- 2 pinches of salt
- 2 oz. of cream cheese
- 2 tsp of psyllium husk ground
- 2 eggs, only whites
- 1/2 cup of almond flour
- 1/4 cup of sunflower seeds
- 1/2 cup of sesame seeds
- 11/2 tsp of baking powder

Instructions

Preheat oven to around 400 degrees F. Mix cream cheese and egg whites in a bowl. Add the rest of the ingredients and mix. Shape squares of the mixture and bake for around 12 minutes by placing them in the pan.

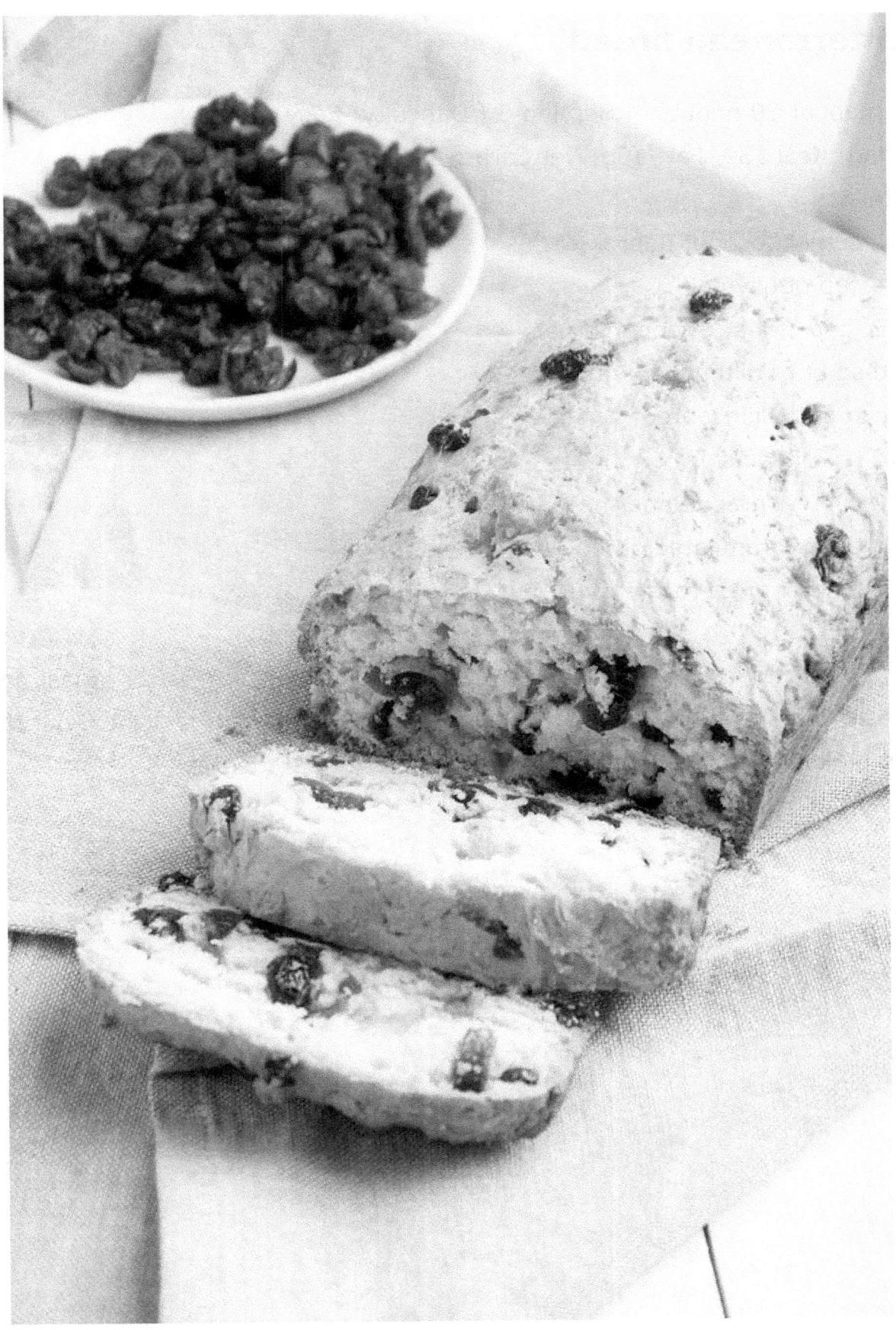

6 Mediterranean bread

(Ready in about 30 minutes | Serving 6 | Difficulty: Easy)

Per serving: Kcal 139, Fat: 12g, Net Carbs: 1g, Protein: 4g

Ingredients

- 1/2 cup of coconut flour
- 1/4 cup of olive oil
- 1/2 tbsp of black peppercorns
- 1 tbsp of psyllium husk ground
- 1 cup of boiling water
- 1/2 tsp of sea salt
- 1/2 cup of shredded parmesan
- 1/4 tsp of granulated garlic
- 1/2 tbsp of dried rosemary

Instructions

Mix dry ingredients in a bowl and add cheese and oil. Add warm water at last and stir. Line baking sheet with parchment paper and flatten dough on it. Roll out the dough to make it thin. Bake for around 25 minutes at 350 degrees F.

7 Parmesan croutons

(Ready in about 1 hour | Serving 8 | Difficulty: Hard)

Per serving: Kcal 259, Fat: 23g, Net Carbs: 1g, Protein: 8g

Ingredients

- 4 oz. of butter
- 1 1/4 cups of almond flour
- 3/4 cup of shredded Parmesan
- 1/3 cup of psyllium husk powder
- 1 tsp of sea salt
- 2 tsp of baking powder
- 2 tsp of cider vinegar
- 3 eggs, only whites
- 1 1/4 cups of boiling water

Instructions

Preheat oven to around 350 degrees F. Add dry ingredients to a bowl and mix. Boil water and add to dry ingredients with egg whites and vinegar. Beat for around 30 seconds. Form flat pieces (8) out of dough and bake for around 40 minutes in the lower rack. Split pieces of bread lengthwise and place on sheet pan face up. Stir parmesan cheese and butter and spread on bread. Broil for around 5 minutes at 450 degrees F.

8 Cloud bread

(Ready in about 30 minutes | Serving 2 | Difficulty: Easy)

Per serving: Kcal 740, Fat: 61g, Net Carbs: 7g, Protein: 37g

Ingredients

- 3 eggs
- 1 pinch of salt
- 4 oz. of cream cheese
- 1/2 tbsp of psyllium husk ground
- 1/4 tsp of cream of tartar
- 1/2 tsp of baking powder

Instructions

Preheat oven to around 300 degrees F. Add egg yolks to one bowl and whites to another. Mix salt in whites and add the rest of the ingredients to yolks. Mix two bowls and place them on a baking tray lined with paper. Spread into circles and bake for around 25 minutes.

9 Garlic focaccia

(Ready in about 25 minutes | Serving 8 | Difficulty: Easy)

Per serving: Kcal 196, Fat: 17g, Net Carbs: 2g, Protein: 8g

Ingredients

Foccacia

- 2 tbsp of cream cheese
- 11/2 cups of shredded cheese mozzarella
- 1 tsp of white wine vinegar
- 1/2 tsp of garlic powder
- 3/4 cup of almond flour
- 1 egg
- 1/2 tsp of salt

Butter

- 1/2 tsp chopped fresh rosemary
- 3 chopped garlic cloves
- 2 oz. of butter
- 1/2 tsp of sea salt

Instructions

Preheat oven to around 400 degrees F. Microwave cream cheese and mozzarella in a bowl. Add the rest of the ingredients and mix. Make the round crust by flattening the dough. Make holes and place them in a tray lined with parchment paper. Bake for around 12 minutes and mix rosemary, garlic, salt and butter in the bowl. Spread on bread and bake for another 10 minutes.

10 Parmesan chips

(Ready in about 10 minutes | Serving 2 | Difficulty: Easy)

Per serving: Kcal 263, Fat: 19g, Net Carbs: 2g, Protein: 17g

Ingredients

- 2 1/2 tbsp of pumpkin seeds
- 1 tbsp of chia seeds
- 3/4 cup of shredded cheese Parmesan
- 2 tbsp of whole flaxseed

Instructions

Preheat oven to around 350 degrees F. Line parchment paper on a baking sheet. Mix seeds and cheese in a bowl. Spoon mixture on a sheet in small mounds. Bake for around 10 minutes.

11 Low-carb bread

(Ready in about 30 minutes | Serving 4 | Difficulty: Easy)

Per serving: Kcal 311, Fat: 14g, Net Carbs: 2g, Protein: 6g

Ingredients

- 4 1/2 oz. of cream cheese
- 3 eggs
- 1 pinch of salt
- 1/2 tsp of baking powder
- 1/2 tbsp of psyllium husk ground
- 1/4 tsp of cream of tartar

Instructions

Separate whites and yolks in two bowls. Add salt to whites and mix. Mix cream cheese with yolks. Add husk powder and baking powder. Fold whites into yolk mixture. Line a baking tray with paper and add dollops of the mixture according to servings. Spread in the form of circles and bake for around 25 minutes at 300 degrees F.

12 Pizza crust

(Ready in about 35 minutes | Serving 4 | Difficulty: Moderate)

Per serving: Kcal 384, Fat: 31g, Net Carbs: 3g, Protein: 17g

Ingredients
- 1 1/4 cups of almond flour
- 1/4 cup of psyllium husk ground
- 1/4 cup of protein powder
- 2 tbsp of parmesan cheese grated
- 1/2 tsp of salt
- 1 1/2 oz. of melted butter
- 1 tbsp of Italian seasoning
- 2 eggs
- 2 tsp of baking powder
- 1 cup of boiling water
- olive oil

Instructions

Preheat oven to around 350 degrees F. Line parchment paper in two baking sheets and coat using oil. Mix dry ingredients in a bowl and stir eggs in it. Add boiling water and mix to form a thick dough. Divide in half and oil gently. Make two balls from the dough. Place on sheets and add parchment paper on the surface. Flatten balls with hands into thin crusts and discard paper. Bake for around 25 minutes. Take out and brush using coconut oil. Broil each side for around 3 minutes. Add toppings and bake for 10 more minutes at 425 degrees F.

13 Zucchini ciabatta

(Ready in about 25 minutes | Serving 4 | Difficulty: Hard)

Per serving: Kcal 409, Fat: 32g, Net Carbs: 7g, Protein: 17g

Ingredients

- 1 lb of zucchini
- 1 cup of almond flour
- sea salt
- 4 eggs
- 1/2 cup of sesame seeds
- 2 tbsp of psyllium husk ground
- 3 tbsp of sunflower seeds
- 1 tbsp of coconut flour
- 11/2 tsp of baking soda
- 1 tbsp of Italian seasoning
- 1/2 tsp of salt

Instructions

Preheat oven to around 400 degrees F. Rinse zucchini and shred finely. Squeeze extra liquid. Beat eggs in zucchini and mix dry ingredients in another bowl. Add to egg mixture and stir. Shape flat elongated pieces of bread and place on a parchment paper-lined baking sheet. Sprinkle sea salt and bake for around 20 minutes.

14 Keto dosa

(Ready in about 15 minutes | Serving 2 | Difficulty: Easy)

Per serving: Kcal 368, Fat: 33g, Net Carbs: 4g, Protein: 13g

Ingredients

- 1/2 cup of almond flour
- 1/2 tsp of coriander seed ground
- 1/2 cup of coconut milk
- 1/2 cup of shredded cheese mozzarella
- 1/2 tsp of ground cumin
- salt

Instructions

Mix everything in a bowl and warm oil in a pan. Pour batter and spread in the pan in a circular shape. Cook until cheese melts. Fold with a spatula once it is done.

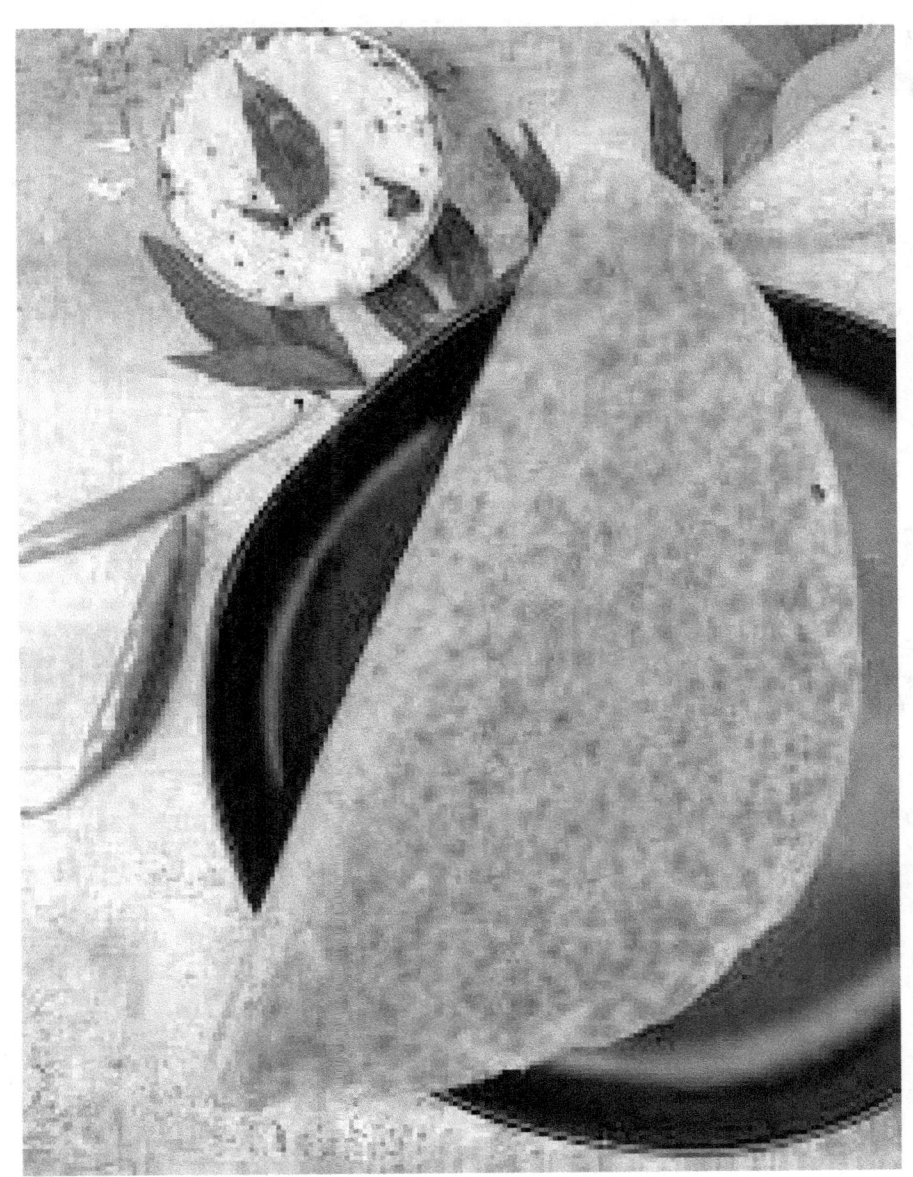

15 Simple keto bread

(Ready in about 1 hour 10 minutes | Serving 6 | Difficulty: Hard)

Per serving: Kcal 311, Fat: 12g, Net Carbs: 2g, Protein: 6g

Ingredients

- 1/3 cup of psyllium husk ground
- 2 tbsp of sesame seeds
- 2 tsp of baking powder
- 11/4 cups of almond flour
- 1 tsp of sea salt
- 2 tsp of cider vinegar
- 1 cup of water
- 3 eggs, only whites

Instructions

Preheat oven to around 350 degrees F. Get a bowl to mix dry ingredients and boil water. Add egg whites and vinegar to the bowl and mix. Add boiling water and whisk into a thick dough. Make six rolls and place them on the baking sheet. Bake for around 60 minutes in the lower rack.

16 Seed crackers

(Ready in about 50 minutes | Serving 30 | Difficulty: Hard)

Per serving: Kcal 60, Fat: 6g, Net Carbs: 1g, Protein: 2g

Ingredients

- 1/3 cup of almond flour
- 1/3 cup of pumpkin seeds unsalted
- 1 tsp of salt
- 1/3 cup of flaxseed
- 1 cup of boiling water
- 1/3 cup of sesame seeds
- 1/3 cup of sunflower seeds unsalted
- 1 tbsp of psyllium husk ground
- 1/4 cup of coconut oil melted

Instructions

Preheat oven to around 300 degrees F. Add dry ingredients to a bowl and mix. Add oil and boiling water and form dough. Line parchment paper on the baking sheet and place dough. Add paper on top and flatten dough. Take the paper on top off and bake for around 45 minutes.

17 Sesame bread

(Ready in about 1 hour | Serving 30 | Difficulty: Hard)

Per serving: Kcal 61, Fat: 5g, Net Carbs: 1g, Protein: 2g

Ingredients

- 1 1/4 cups of sesame seeds
- 1/2 cup of cheddar cheese shredded
- 1/2 cup of sunflower seeds
- 1 tbsp of psyllium husk ground
- 2 eggs
- 1/2 cup of water
- 1/4 tsp of salt

Instructions

Preheat oven to around 350 degrees F. Line parchment paper in the baking sheet and mix everything in a bowl. Spread mixture on paper and sprinkle with salt. Bake for around 20 minutes. Take out and cut into the shape of your preference. Now bake for around 40 minutes at 275 degrees F.

18 Holiday bread

(Ready in about 1 hour | Serving 22 | Difficulty: Hard)

Per serving: Kcal 151, Fat: 12g, Net Carbs: 2g, Protein: 5g

Ingredients

- 2 cups of almond flour
- 1/3 cup of sesame seeds
- 1/2 cup of coconut flour
- 1 cup of sour cream
- 1/3 cup of flaxseed
- 1 tbsp of baking powder
- 1/4 cup of psyllium husk ground
- 3/4 tbsp of ground cloves
- 1/2 tbsp of fennel seeds
- 1/2 tbsp of orange peel ground
- 1 tsp of anise seeds
- 1 tsp of salt
- 1 tsp of ground cardamom
- 6 eggs
- 3 oz. of cream cheese

Instructions

Preheat the oven to 400 degrees F. Add dry ingredients to a bowl and mix. Mix cream cheese, eggs and sour cream in another bowl. Add to dry mixture and stir. Line a pan with parchment paper and pour the mixture on it. Bake for around 60 minutes.

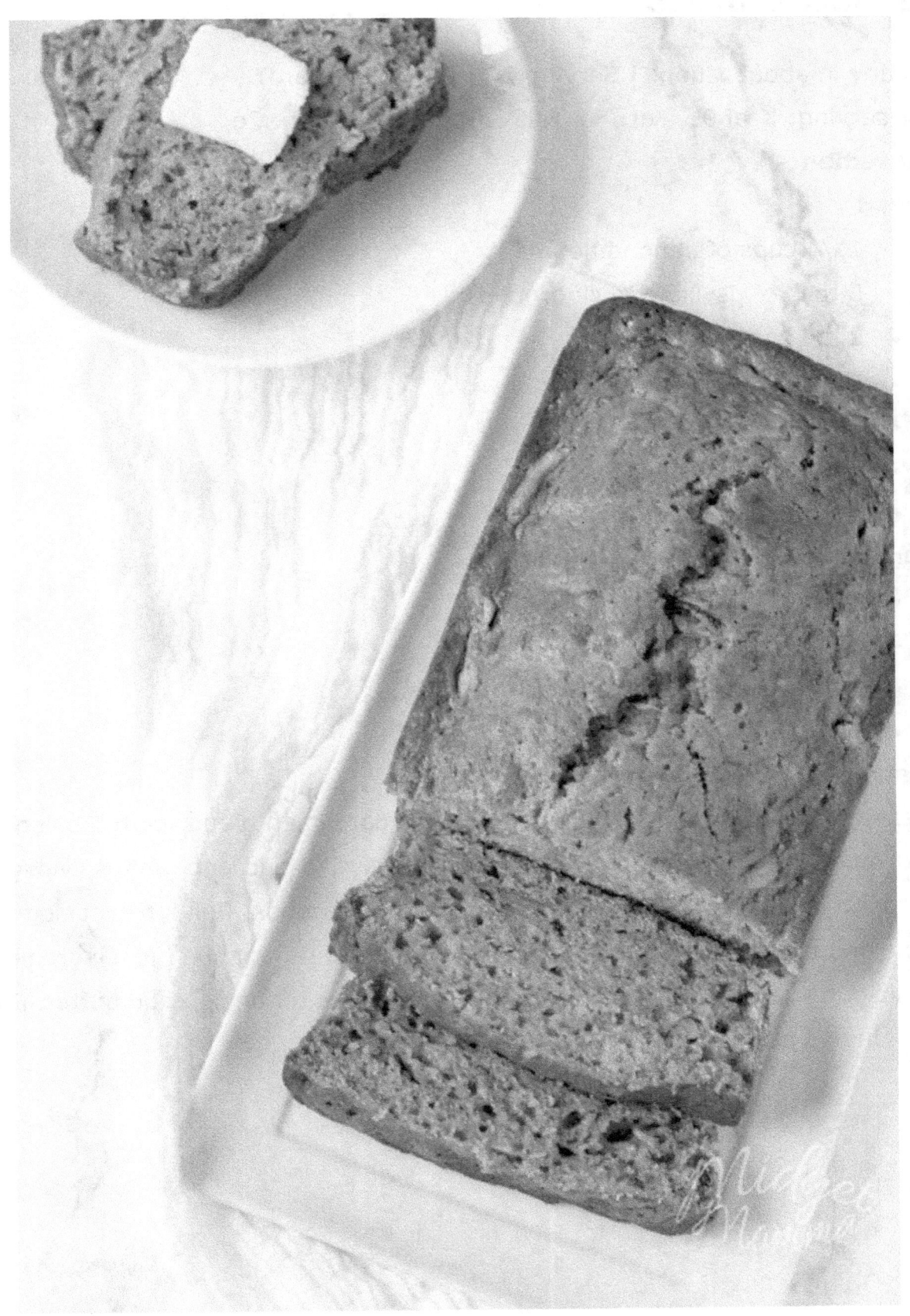

19 Butter bread

(Ready in about 1 hour | Serving 20 | Difficulty: Hard)

Per serving: Kcal 91, Fat: 8g, Net Carbs: 1g, Protein: 2g

Ingredients

Bread

- 11/4 cups of almond flour
- 5 tbsp of psyllium husk ground
- 2 tsp of baking powder
- 1 tsp of sea salt
- 1 cup of water
- 2 tsp of cider vinegar
- 3 eggs, only whites

Garlic butter

- 4 oz. of butter
- 1 minced garlic clove
- 2 tbsp chopped fresh parsley
- 1/2 tsp of salt

Instructions

Preheat oven to around 350 degrees F. Line parchment paper on the baking sheet and mix dry ingredients in a bowl. Boil water and add egg whites, vinegar and water to dry ingredients. Whisk for around 30 seconds. Roll into hot dog-shaped buns and place them on a sheet. Bake for around 40 minutes. Mix ingredients for garlic butter and refrigerate. Cut buns from the center and spread butter. Bake for 15 minutes at 425 degrees F.

20 Bread twists

(Ready in about 25 minutes | Serving 10 | Difficulty: Easy)

Per serving: Kcal 181, Fat: 16g, Net Carbs: 1g, Protein: 7g

Ingredients

- 1/2 cup of almond flour
- 1/2 tsp of salt
- 1/4 cup of green pesto
- 1/4 cup of coconut flour
- 1 tsp of baking powder
- 2 oz. of butter
- 1 beaten egg
- 12/3 cups of shredded cheese mozzarella
- 1 beaten egg

Instructions

Preheat oven to around 350 degrees F. Add dry ingredients to a bowl and mix. Whisk eggs in a mixture and use a pot to melt cheese and butter. Add to bowl and make a firm dough by mixing. Place parchment paper and add dough to it. Form a rectangle with a rolling pin. Add pesto over dough and dice into strips(1 inch approx.). Twist and place on a parchment paper-lined baking sheet. Bake for around 20 minutes.

21 French toast

(Ready in about 10 minutes | Serving 2 | Difficulty: Easy)

Per serving: Kcal 408, Fat: 37g, Net Carbs: 3g, Protein: 15g

Ingredients

Bread

- 2 tbsp of almond flour
- 2 tbsp of whipping cream
- 1 tsp of butter
- 2 tbsp of coconut flour
- 1 pinch of salt
- 1 1/2 tsp of baking powder
- 2 eggs

Batter

- 1 pinch of salt
- 2 tbsp of whipping cream
- 2 eggs
- 1/2 tsp of ground cinnamon
- 2 tbsp of butter

Instructions

Coat a glass dish with butter. Mix dry ingredients and break an egg. Stir and microwave for around 2 minutes. Take out of dish and dice in two pieces. Mix the rest of the ingredients in a bowl and pour on slices. Fry in butter and enjoy.

22 Soft tortillas

(Ready in about 20 minutes | Serving 6 | Difficulty: Easy)

Per serving: Kcal 236, Fat: 21g, Net Carbs: 1g, Protein: 5g

Ingredients

- 1/4 tsp of baking soda
- 11/2 cups of hot water
- 1 cup of coconut flour
- 1/2 tsp of salt
- 1/2 cup of avocado oil
- 1/4 cup of psyllium husk ground
- 3 egg whites

Instructions

Warm oil in a pan and mix baking soda, salt and coconut flour in a bowl. Whisk husk and drizzle oil. Fold in whites and add hot water, around 1/2 cup at once. Combine to form dough and shape into 12 balls. Place balls between parchment and flatten using a tortilla press. Toast each side for around 3 minutes.

23 Nut-free bread

(Ready in about 40 minutes | Serving 20 | Difficulty: Moderate)

Per serving: Kcal 109, Fat: 9g, Net Carbs: 1g, Protein: 6g

Ingredients

- 1 tbsp melted butter
- 6 eggs
- 1 oz. of cream cheese
- 3 cups of shredded cheese
- 2 tbsp of psyllium husk ground
- 1/2 cup of oat fiber
- 3 tsp of baking powder
- 1/2 tsp of salt

Topping

- 2 tbsp of poppy seeds
- 3 tbsp of sesame seeds

Instructions

Preheat oven to around 360 degrees F. Whisk eggs and add rest of ingredients in a bowl except butter. Coat a pan using butter and spread dough using a spatula. Sprinkle seeds on the dough and bake for around 35 minutes.

24 Fluffy bread

(Ready in about 1 hour 20 minutes | Serving 18 | Difficulty: Hard)

Per serving: Kcal 82, Fat: 7g, Net Carbs: 3g, Protein: 4g

Ingredients

- 1 cup of Almond Flour
- 1/3 cup of Butter
- 2 tsp of baking powder Gluten-free
- 1/4 cup of Coconut Flour
- 1/4 tsp of Sea salt
- 12 Egg whites

Instructions

Preheat oven to around 325 degrees F. Line parchment paper on a pan and add all the ingredients except tartar and eggs to the processor. Pulse and beat egg whites and tartar in a bowl using a hand mixer. Add half amount of whites to the processor and pulse. Transfer to bowl with rest of whites. Fold gently and place in pan. Bake for around 40 minutes. Bake for another 30 minutes after covering with foil.

25 90 Seconds Bread

(Ready in about 2 minutes | Serving 1 | Difficulty: Easy)

Per serving: Kcal 220, Fat: 21g, Net Carbs: 4g, Protein: 4g

Ingredients

- 1 tbsp of coconut flour
- 1 egg
- 1 tbsp of butter
- 1/2 tsp of baking powder double acting

Instructions

Add butter to a bowl and microwave. Mix the rest of the ingredients in butter and beat. Microwave for around 2 minutes and slice in two parts. Preheat oven to around 375 degrees F and bake for around 12 minutes.

26 Almond Flour Bread

(Ready in about 50 minutes | Serving 12 | Difficulty: Hard)

Per serving: Kcal 156, Fat: 14.2g, Net Carbs: 3.6g, Protein: 5.2g

Ingredients

- 2 whites of eggs
- pinch of salt
- 2 cups almond flour
- 2 eggs, yolks & whites
- 1/4 cup of butter melted
- 1 1/2 tsp of baking powder
- 4 tbsp of psyllium husks
- 1/2 tsp of xanthan gum
- 1/2 cup of warm water

Instructions

Preheat oven to around 350 degrees F. Break 2 eggs and 2 whites and beat. Add the rest of the ingredients and make a smooth dough by blending. Fill the baking tin and bake for around 45 minutes.

27 Plain Bread

(Ready in about 1 hour | Serving 12 | Difficulty: Hard)

Per serving: Kcal 247, Fat: 22.8g, Net Carbs: 4.9g, Protein: 7.7g

Ingredients

- 7 eggs
- cooking spray
- 1/2tsp of xanthan gum
- 1/2 cup melted butter
- 2 cups of almond flour blanched
- 2 tbsp of olive oil
- 1 tsp of baking powder
- 1/2tsp of sea salt

Instructions

Preheat oven to around 350 degrees F. Coat a pan using cooking spray and break and beat eggs in a bowl. Add butter and oil and mix. Mix the rest of the ingredients in another bowl. Add to eggs and mix. Pour in pan and bake for around 45 minutes.

28 Fathead Bread

(Ready in about 55 minutes | Serving 4 | Difficulty: Hard)

Per serving: Kcal 240, Fat: 19.4g, Net Carbs: 4.2g, Protein: 13.5g

Ingredients

- 3/4 cup of shredded cheese mozzarella
- 1 egg
- 2 ounces of cream cheese
- 1/3 cup of almond flour
- 1/4tsp of garlic powder
- 2 tsp of baking powder
- 1/2 cup of shredded cheese Cheddar

Instructions

Microwave cream cheese and mozzarella in a bowl for around 20 seconds. Beat eggs in a bowl and add the rest of the ingredients. Add mozzarella mixture and mix. Transfer to plastic wrap and wrap over dough. Form a ball and place it in the fridge for around 30 minutes. Preheat oven to around 425 degrees F and oil a parchment paper-lined baking sheet. Take the dough out and remove the wrap. Make 4 pieces and roll each into the shape of a ball. Cut in half and place on sheet. Bake for around 12 minutes.

29 Bread Rolls

(Ready in about 1 hour 5 minutes | Serving 8 | Difficulty: Hard)

Per serving: Kcal 166, Fat: 12g, Net Carbs: 10g, Protein: 6.8g

Ingredients

- cooking spray
- 5 tbsp of psyllium husk
- 2 tbsp of sesame seeds
- 1 1/2 cups of almond flour blanched
- 1 tsp of sea salt
- 3 eggs, only whites
- 1 cup of boiling water
- 2 tsp of white vinegar

Instructions

Preheat oven to around 350 degrees F. Oil a baking sheet using cooking spray. Add the rest of the ingredients to a bowl and mix using an electric mixer to form a dough. Make 8 rolls from the dough and place them on a sheet. Sprinkle seeds and bake for around 55 minutes.

30 Simple and Easy Bread

(Ready in about 1 hour 10 minutes | Serving 1 | Difficulty: Hard)

Per serving: Kcal 450, Fat: 40g, Net Carbs: 10g, Protein: 19g

Ingredients

- 6 eggs
- 1 tbsp of baking powder
- 1/4 cup of melted butter
- 1/2 tsp of cream of tartar
- 1 1/2 cup of finely ground almond flour
- 1/2 tsp of kosher salt

Instructions

Preheat oven to around 375 degrees F. Line parchment paper in a pan and separate egg yolks and whites. Combine whites with tartar in a bowl and beat yolk with the rest of the ingredients in another bowl. Fold in whites and transfer to pan. Bake for around 30 minutes.

31 Gluten-free Bread

(Ready in about 1 hour 15 minutes | Serving 10 | Difficulty: Hard)

Per serving: Kcal 53, Fat: 3g, Net Carbs: 4g, Protein: 2g

Ingredients

- 1 1/4 cups of almond flour
- 2 tbsp of sesame seeds
- 2 tsp of baking powder
- 5 tbsp of psyllium husk ground
- 1 tsp of salt
- 1 cup of boiling water
- 2 tsp of apple cider vinegar
- 3 eggs, only whites

Instructions

Preheat oven to around 350 degrees F. Line parchment paper in loaf tin after coating with butter. Combine husk, salt, almond flour and baking powder in a bowl. Add cider vinegar and egg whites to dry ingredients and mix using an electric mixer. Add boiling water slowly and mix. A dough will form. Transfer to the tin and sprinkle seeds. Bake for around 60 minutes.

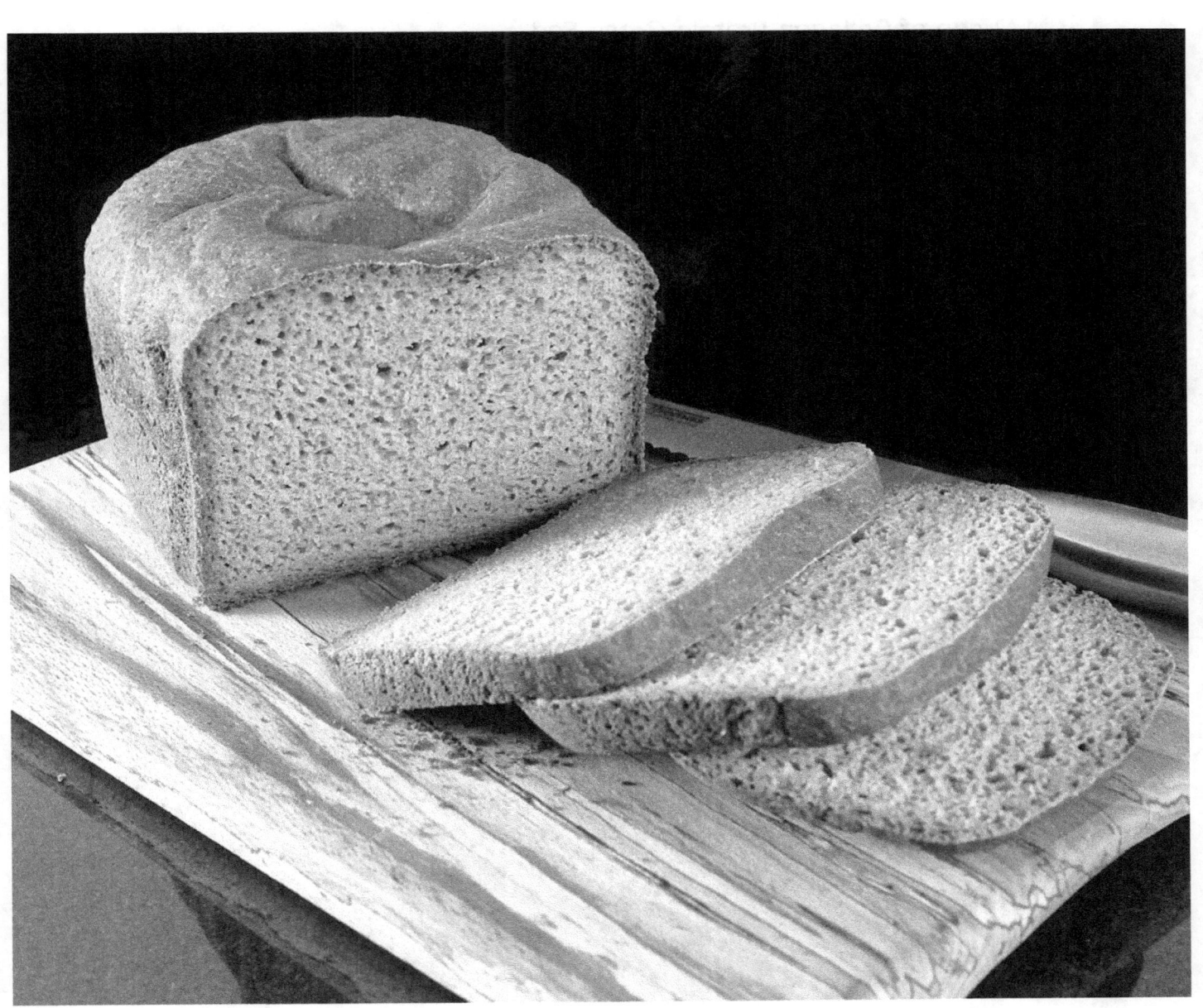

32 Collagen Bread

(Ready in about 1 hour 50 minutes | Serving 12 | Difficulty: Hard)

Per serving: Kcal 311, Fat: 5g, Net Carbs: 1g, Protein: 7g

Ingredients

- 1/2 cup of Collagen Protein Grass-Fed
- 1 tsp of xanthan gum
- 6 tbsp of almond flour
- 5 separated eggs, pastured
- 1 tbsp of coconut oil unflavored
- 1 tsp of baking powder aluminum-free
- Pinch of Himalayan salt

Instructions

Preheat oven to around 325 degrees F. Oil a loaf dish and beat egg whites in a bowl. Mix dry ingredients in another bowl. Mix yolks, coconut oil and wet ingredients in another bowl. Add both mixtures to whites and beat. Pour into the dish and bake for around 40 minutes.

33 Coconut Bread

(Ready in about 1 hour 10 minutes | Serving 10 | Difficulty: Hard)

Per serving: Kcal 318, Fat: 17g, Net Carbs: 9g, Protein: 12g

Ingredients

- 1/2 cup coconut flour
- 1/4 cup of coconut oil
- 1/4 tsp of baking soda
- 1/4 tsp of salt
- 6 eggs
- 1/4 of almond milk unsweetened

Instructions

Preheat your oven to around 350 degrees F. Line parchment paper in a pan and combine salt, soda and coconut flour in a bowl. Mix oil, milk and eggs in another bowl. Incorporate both mixtures and pour in pan. Bake for around 50 minutes.

34 Macadamia Bread

(Ready in about 35 minutes | Serving 10 | Difficulty: Moderate)

Per serving: Kcal 151, Fat: 14g, Net Carbs: 4g, Protein: 5g

Ingredients

- 5 oz of macadamia nuts
- 1/2 tsp of apple cider vinegar
- 1/4 cup of coconut flour
- 5 eggs
- 1/2 tsp of baking soda

Instructions

Preheat oven to around 350 degrees F. Pulse nuts in processor and add eggs, and pulse again. Add rest of ingredients and pulse to incorporate thoroughly. Oil a pan and pour the mixture, and bake for around 40 minutes.

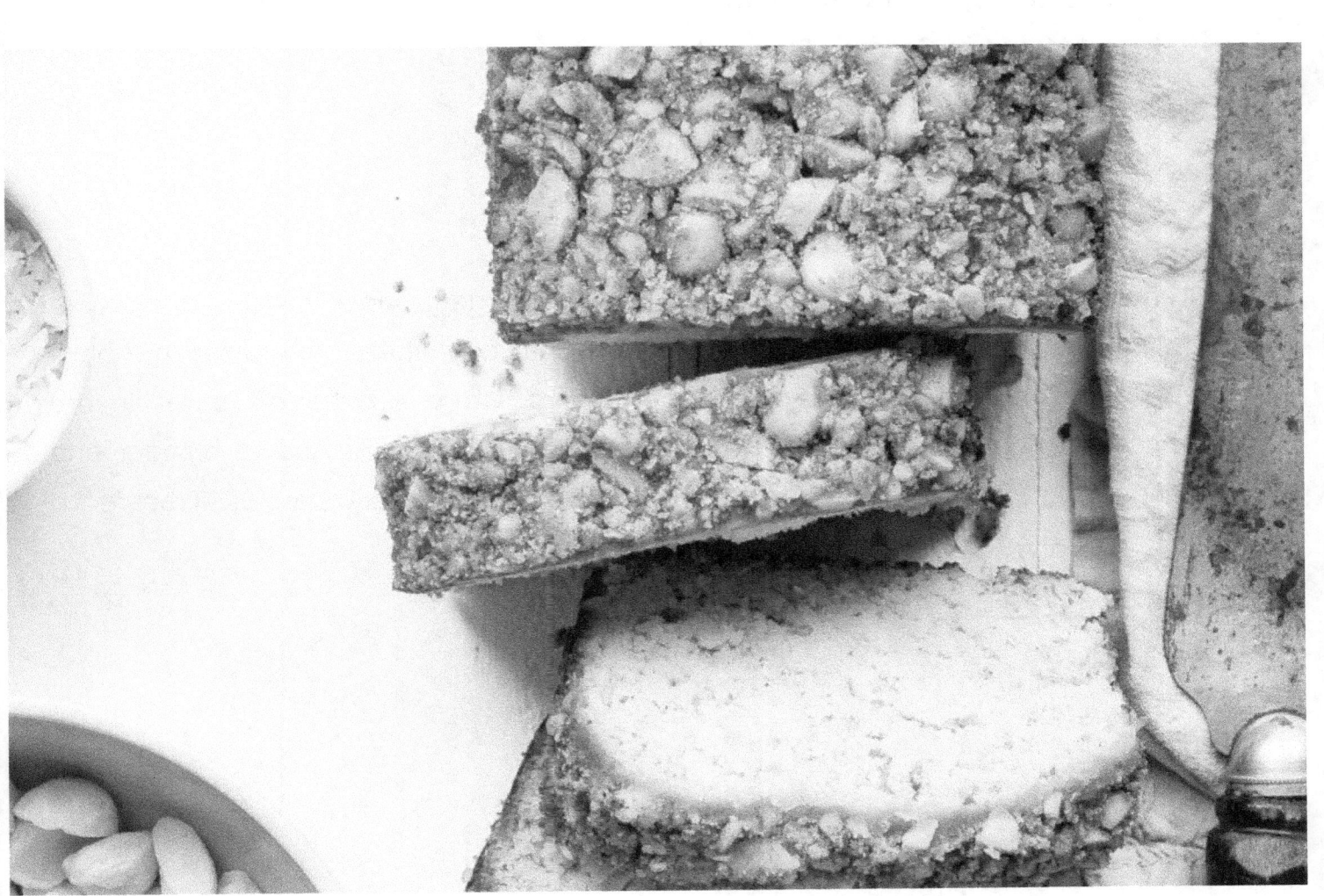

35 Cauliflower Bread

(Ready in about 1 hour 18 minutes | Serving 6 | Difficulty: Hard)

Per serving: Kcal 108, Fat: 8g, Net Carbs: 8g, Protein: 6g

Ingredients

- 3 cups of riced cauliflower
- 1 tbsp chopped fresh rosemary
- 1 1/4 cup of Coconut Flour Wholesome
- 10 separated Egg
- 1 1/2 tbsp of baking powder Gluten-free
- 1 tbsp chopped fresh parsley

Instructions

Preheat oven to around 350 degrees F. Line parchment paper in a pan and steam cauliflower in the microwave until it is soft. Beat egg whites and tartar in a bowl with a mixer. Add the rest of the ingredients with a quarter of whites in the processor. Squeeze cauliflower in a kitchen towel to dry it. Add to blender and pulse. Add rest of whites and pulse. Fold in the rosemary and parsley. Transfer to pan and bake for around 50 minutes.

36 Keto Tortillas

(Ready in about 15 minutes | Serving 8 | Difficulty: Easy)

Per serving: Kcal 89, Fat: 6g, Net Carbs: 4g, Protein: 3g

Ingredients

- 96 g of almond flour
- 3 tsp of water
- 2 tsp of xanthan gum
- 24 g of coconut flour
- 1 tsp of baking powder
- 2 tsp of apple cider vinegar
- 1/4 tsp of kosher salt
- 1 beaten egg

Instructions

Break eggs in a bowl and whisk. Add rest of ingredients except cider vinegar in processor and blend. Add cider vinegar while the blender is running. Once it is uniformly distributed, add eggs and water. Once a ball forms from the dough, stop. Wrap using cling film and through plastic, knead for around 1 minute. Warm a pan and form eight balls of 1 inch. Roll out balls in two parchment papers. Place in pan and cook for around 6 seconds. Flip and cook until each side is a bit golden.

37 Buttery Flatbread

(Ready in about 7 minutes | Serving 2 | Difficulty: Easy)

Per serving: Kcal 232, Fat: 19g, Net Carbs: 9g, Protein: 9g

Ingredients

- 1 cup of Almond Flour
- 1 tbsp of Oil
- 2 tsp of Xanthan Gum
- 2 tbsp of Coconut Flour
- 1/2 tsp of Baking Powder
- 1 Egg plus 1 Egg White
- 1/2 tsp of Falk Salt
- 1 tbsp of Water
- 1 tbsp of melted Butter

Instructions

Mix dry ingredients in a bowl. Add eggs to flour and mix. Add water and work with dough, so moisture is absorbed. Make 4 parts of dough and press using cling wrap. Warm oil in the pan and fry each side of bread for around 1 minute. Brush butter on top and garnish using parsley and salt.

38 Gluten-Free Biscuits

(Ready in about 30 minutes | Serving 6 | Difficulty: Easy)

Per serving: Kcal 290, Fat: 30g, Net Carbs: 8g, Protein: 7g

Ingredients

- 1 egg
- 2 tsp. of apple vinegar
- 77 g of sour cream
- 2 tbsp of water
- 96 g of almond flour
- 1 tbsp of apple cider vinegar
- 63 g of flaxseed meal golden
- 20 g of whey protein
- 21 g of coconut flour
- 3 1/2 tsp of baking powder
- 1/2 tsp of kosher salt
- 1 tsp of xanthan gum
- 112 g of organic butter grass-fed

Instructions

Preheat your oven to around 450 degrees F. Line parchment paper in a tray. Mix eggs, water, apple vinegar and sour cream in a bowl. Add rest of ingredients except butter in blender and pulse. Add butter and blend again. Pour bowl mixture and blend until incorporated. Make 6 rounds from dough and place in the tray. Brush butter and place in oven. Bake for around 20 minutes.

39 Cauliflower Buns

(Ready in about 45 minutes | Serving 6 | Difficulty: Hard)

Per serving: Kcal 43, Fat: 1.9g, Net Carbs: 3.5g, Protein: 3.3g

Ingredients

- 2 cups of cauliflower rice
- 2 tbsp of coconut flour
- 2 beaten eggs
- 1/4 tsp of ground turmeric
- 1/4 tsp of black pepper ground
- 1/2 tsp of sea salt

Instructions

Preheat your oven to around 400 degrees F. Line parchment paper on the baking sheet. Mix everything in a bowl and make six buns from the batter. Place on sheet and bake for around 30 minutes.

40 Low Carb Biscuits

(Ready in about 25 minutes | Serving 12 | Difficulty: Easy)

Per serving: Kcal 164, Fat: 15g, Net Carbs: 4g, Protein: 5g

Ingredients

- 1/3 cup of Butter
- 2 cups of Blanched Wholesome Yum Almond Flour
- 1/2 tsp of Sea salt
- 2 tsp of baking powder Gluten-free
- 2 whisked egg

Instructions

Preheat oven to around 350 degrees F. Line parchment paper on the baking sheet. Add all the ingredients to a bowl and whisk. Scoop on the sheet in the amount of tbsp. Form biscuit shapes and bake for around 15 minutes.

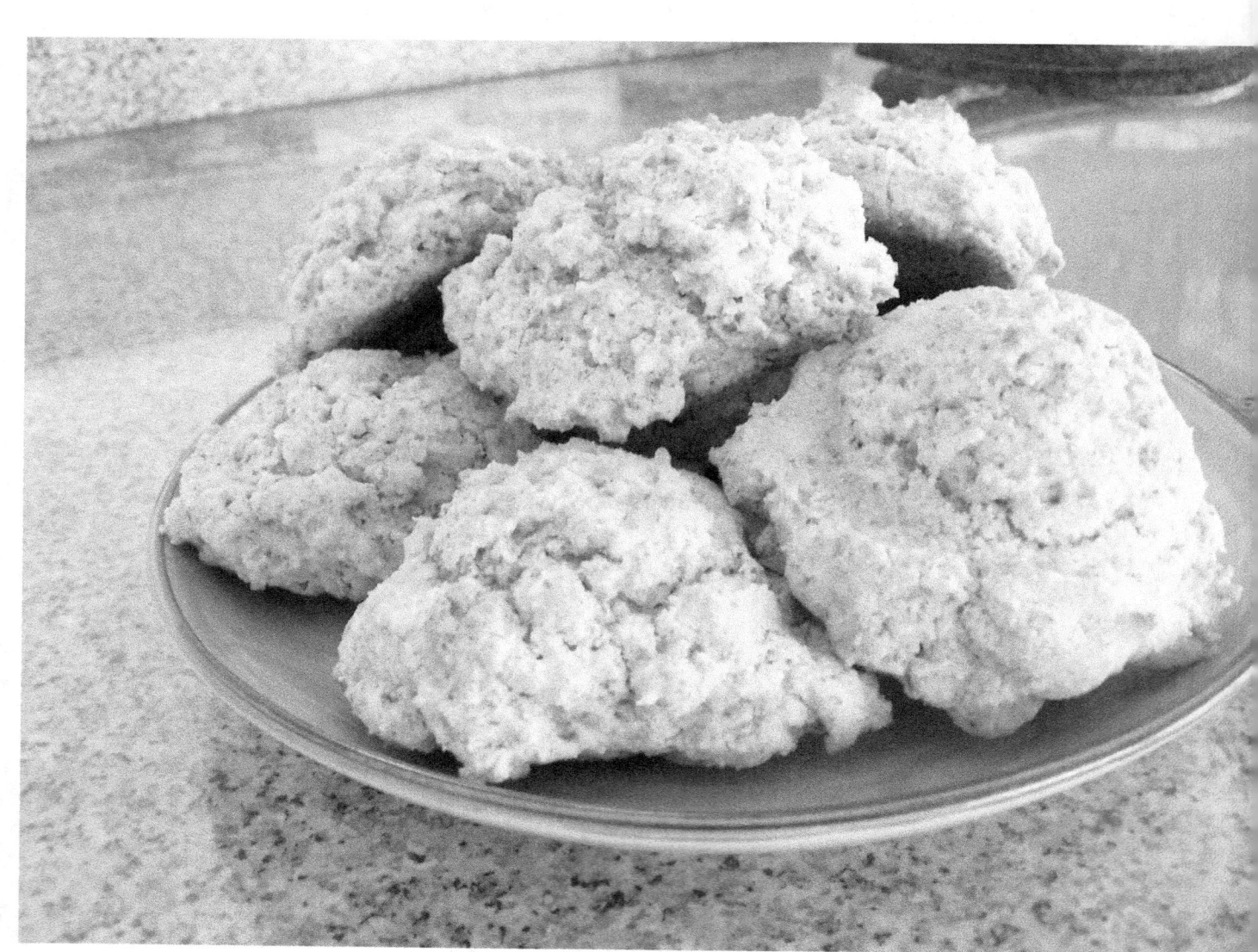

41 Pizza Crust

(Ready in about 10 minutes | Serving 4| Difficulty: Easy)

Per serving: Kcal 125, Fat: 10g, Net Carbs: 6g, Protein: 8g

Ingredients
- 1 tbsp of coconut flour
- 8 egg whites
- 1/2 tsp of baking powder
- 1/4 cup of sifted coconut flour
- Pepper, salt and Italian spices

Pizza sauce
- 1 tsp of dried basil
- 2 cloves of garlic crushed
- 1/2 cup of tomato sauce
- 1/4 tsp of sea salt

Instructions

Whisk egg in a bowl and add coconut flour. Whisk and add mixed spices and baking powder and keep whisking until fully incorporated. Warm a pan after oiling it lightly. Pour mixture into the pan and cook for around 4 minutes. Flip and cook for 2 more minutes. Dust with coconut flour. Combine sauce ingredients in a bowl and spread on crust.

42 Zucchini Bread

(Ready in about 1 hour 20 minutes | Serving 16 | Difficulty: Hard)

Per serving: Kcal 200, Fat: 17g, Net Carbs: 2.6g, Protein: 6g

Ingredients

- 3 eggs
- 1 tsp of vanilla extract
- 1/2cup of olive oil
- 2 1/2cups of almond flour
- 1 cup of grated zucchini
- 1/2tsp of salt
- 1 1/2 cups of erythritol
- 1 1/2tsp of baking powder
- 1 tsp of ground cinnamon
- 1/2tsp of nutmeg
- 1/4tsp of ground ginger
- 1/2cup of chopped walnuts

Instructions

Preheat your oven to around 350 degrees F. Mix oil, eggs and vanilla in a bowl. Mix erythritol, baking powder, salt, nutmeg, almond flour, ginger and cinnamon in another bowl. Squeeze zucchini in a paper towel and add to eggs. Add dry ingredients to the egg and blend. Spray a pan using cooking spray and spoon mixture. Add walnuts and press with a spatula. Bake for around 70 minutes.

43 Blueberry Muffin Bread

(Ready in about 1 hour | Serving 12 | Difficulty: Hard)

Per serving: Kcal 156, Fat: 13g, Net Carbs: 4g, Protein: 5g

Ingredients

- 1/4 cup of butter
- 1/2 cup of almond butter
- 5 eggs
- 1/2 cup of almond flour
- 2 tsp of baking powder
- 1/2 tsp of salt
- 1/2 cup of almond milk
- 1/2 cup of blueberries

Instructions

Preheat the oven to around 350 degrees F. Melt butter and nut butter in a bowl and stir. Mix baking powder, salt and almond flour in another bowl and pour butter mixture. Stir and take another bowl to mix eggs and almond milk. Pour in flour and butter mixture and stir. Add blueberries and stir. Line parchment paper in the pan and oil it. Pour batter and bake for around 45 minutes.

44 Cranberry Bread

(Ready in about 1 hour 25 minutes | Serving 12 | Difficulty: Hard)

Per serving: Kcal 175, Fat: 14g, Net Carbs: 8g, Protein: 7g

Ingredients

- 1 1/2 cups of almond flour
- 1/2 cup of white sweetener
- 1/2 cup of almond milk unsweetened
- 1/2 cup of coconut flour
- 1/2tsp of 30% extract monk fruit
- 1 1/2tsp of baking powder
- 1 tbsp of orange peel dried
- 1/2tsp of baking soda
- 1/2tsp of ground cinnamon
- 1/2tsp of xanthan gum
- 1/2tsp of salt
- 1/4 cup of butter melted unsalted
- 1/4tsp of ground nutmeg
- 6 eggs
- 6 ounces of cranberries

Instructions

Preheat oven to around 325 degrees F. Oil a pan and line using parchment paper. Mix everything except butter, egg and almond milk in a bowl. Mix them in a separate bowl. Add to dry ingredients and whisk. Fold the mixture in cranberries and pour in a pan. Bake for around 1 hour.

45 Fluffy Buns

(Ready in about 30 minutes | Serving 4 | Difficulty: Easy)

Per serving: Kcal 109, Fat: 12.5g, Net Carbs: 2.3g, Protein: 7.3g

Ingredients

- 1 egg
- 1 tsp of baking powder
- 3 eggs, only whites
- 1/4 cup of hot water
- 1/4 cup of coconut flour
- 1/4 cup of almond flour
- 1 tbsp of psyllium husk ground
- Sesame seeds

Instructions

Preheat oven to around 356 F and mix dry ingredients in a bowl. Add everything to the blender and blend for around 20 seconds. Make four portions from dough and shape buns. Place on sheet and sprinkle seeds on top. Bake for around 25 minutes.

46 Ultimate Buns

(Ready in about 1 hour | Serving 1 | Difficulty: Hard)

Per serving: Kcal 208, Fat: 15.2g, Net Carbs: 4.2g, Protein: 10.1g

Dry ingredients

- 2/3 cup of psyllium husks ground
- 1 1/2 cup of almond flour
- 1/2 cup of coconut flour
- 5 tbsp of sesame seeds2 tsp of garlic powder
- 1/2 cup of flax meal
- 2 tsp of onion powder
- 1 tsp of baking soda
- 2 tsp of cream of tartar
- 1 tsp of Himalayan salt

Wet ingredients

- 2 eggs
- 6 egg whites
- 2 cups of water

Instructions

Preheat oven to around 350 degrees F. Add dry ingredients except for sesame seeds and mix. Add eggs and mix. Make buns with a spoon. Line a tray using parchment paper and place buns. Top with seeds and bake for around 55 minutes.

47 Dinner Rolls

(Ready in about 15 minutes | Serving 6 | Difficulty: Easy)

Per serving: Kcal 219, Fat: 18g, Net Carbs: 5.6g, Protein: 16g10.7g

Ingredients

- 1 Cup of Mozzarella, shredded
- 1 Cup of Almond Flour
- 1 oz of Cream Cheese
- 1/4 Cup of Flax Seed Ground
- 1/2 Tsp of Baking Soda
- 1 egg

Instructions

Preheat the oven to around 400 degrees F. Line parchment paper on the baking sheet. Microwave mozzarella and cream cheese in a bowl. Stir and add eggs. Combine baking soda, flax and almond flour in another bowl. Add egg mixture and cheese to this mixture. Make 6 balls from the dough. Place on sheet and bake for around 12 minutes.

48 Bagel Scones

(Ready in about 40 minutes | Serving 12 | Difficulty: Moderate)

Per serving: Kcal 161, Fat: 13.5g, Net Carbs: 6.5g, Protein: 5.7g

Ingredients

- 2 cups of almond flour
- 1 tbsp of baking powder
- 1/4 cup of coconut flour
- 1/2 tsp of garlic powder
- 2 eggs
- 1/4 tsp of salt
- 1/4 cup of whipping cream
- 2 tbsp of Bagel Seasoning
- 1 tbsp of butter melted

Instructions

Preheat the oven to around 325 degrees F. Line parchment paper on the baking sheet and oil it gently. Mix everything except bagel seasoning, whipping cream and egg in a bowl. Then stir whipping cream and egg until you get a dough. Place on sheet and shape into a rectangle roughly. Make 6 squares with a knife and cut diagonally each to make two triangles. Sprinkle with bagel seasoning and bake for around 25 minutes.

49 Avocado bread

(Ready in about 1 hour 35 minutes | Serving 9 | Difficulty: Hard)

Per serving: Kcal 214, Fat: 19.1g, Net Carbs: 4.5g, Protein: 10.3g

Ingredients

- 1 cup of almond flour
- 2 tbsp of Swerve Sweetener
- 1/3 cup of whey protein
- 2 tsp of baking powder
- 3 eggs, separated
- 1/2 tsp of salt
- 1 large egg
- 2 tbsp of water
- 3 tbsp of avocado oil
- 1/2 tsp of cream of tartar

Instructions

Preheat oven to around 325 degrees F and line parchment paper in the pan. Mix dry ingredients in one bowl and wet ingredients except tartar and whites in a separate bowl. Add egg mixture to dry ingredients and whisk to combine. Beat whites and tartar in another bowl and fold whites in the batter. Pour batter into the pan and cook for around 50 minutes.

50 Croissants

(Ready in about 50 minutes | Serving 8 | Difficulty: Hard)

Per serving: Kcal 141, Fat: 9.6g, Net Carbs: 4.6g, Protein: 8.4g

Ingredients

- 1 tbsp melted butter
- 1/4 cup of coconut flour
- 1/2 tsp of xanthan gum
- 2 tbsp of Sweetener
- 1 tsp of baking powder
- 1 egg
- 6 ounces of mozzarella
- 1/3 tbsp of almond paste
- 1 tbsp of sliced almonds

Instructions

Preheat oven to around 400 degrees F. Line a baking sheet and whisk coconut flour, xantham gum, baking powder and sweetener in a bowl. Melt cheese in the microwave for around 30 seconds. Knead after stirring in the egg and flour mixture in the bowl with a spatula. Pour on the sheet and cover with parchment paper. Roll into a circle of 12 inches. Take 1.5 tbsp of almond paste and shape a thin log of length around 3 inches. Position at the wide end of 1 wedge and fold the dough around almond paste tightly. Pinch to seal and repeat with the rest of the dough. Curve ends of dough to make a crescent shape. Add sliced almonds and bake for around 25 minutes after turning the temperature to 350 degrees F. Dust using sweetener.

51 Gluten-Free Bagels

(Ready in about 30 minutes | Serving 6 | Difficulty: Easy)

Per serving: Kcal 364, Fat: 27.9g, Sodium 919.8mg, Protein: 20.9g

Ingredients

- 1 tbsp. baking powder, gluten-free
- 1 ½ cups of almond flour
- 2 eggs
- 1 tsp. garlic salt
- 2 oz. cream cheese, cubed
- 2 ½ cups of shredded mozzarella cheese

Instructions

- Preheat oven to 400 degrees Fahrenheit. Using parchment paper, line the baking sheet.
- In a mixing bowl, add the baking powder, garlic salt, and almond flour.
- In the microwave-safe bowl, mix mozzarella and cream cheese. Microwave for one minute, then remove and mix. Microwave for another minute, then take it off and stir until all is well combined. Working fast, stir the eggs and flour mixture into melted cheese mixture. Knead the dough by hand until it becomes a sticky dough. Continue kneading and pressing the dough for approximately two minutes or until it is fully uniform.
- The dough can be divided into six equal bits. Roll each one into the long log, then push the ends together to form a bagel shape and put it on the baking sheet that has been prepared.
- For ten to fourteen minutes in the preheated oven, bake till the bagels are golden.

52 Fluffy Keto Pancakes

(Ready in about 10 minutes | Serving 4 | Difficulty: Easy)
Per serving: Kcal 383, Fat: 32.2g, Sodium 842.3mg, Protein: 15.3g

Ingredients
- ¼ cup of coconut flour
- 1 cup of almond flour
- 2 tbsp. natural sweetener, low-calorie
- 1 tsp. baking powder
- 1 tsp. salt
- ½ tsp. ground cinnamon
- ¼ cup of heavy whipping cream, at room temp.
- 6 eggs, at room temp.
- 1 tsp. vanilla extract
- 2 tbsp. melted butter

Directions
- In a mixing bowl, add coconut flour, almond flour, salt, sweetener, cinnamon, and baking powder. Slowly whisk in the heavy cream, eggs, vanilla extract, and butter till just mixed.
- Over medium-high flame, gently oil a griddle. Cook till the bubbles form and the sides are dry, three to four minutes, by dropping batter by big spoonfuls onto griddle. Cook for two or three minutes on the other hand, until browned. Continue with the remaining batter.
- Cholesterol 281.2mg

53 High Protein Bread

(Ready in about 2hrs 40 mins | Serving 10 | Difficulty: Medium)
Per serving: Kcal 137, Fat: 2.4g, Sodium 235mg, Protein: 6.5g

Ingredients
- 2 tsp dry yeast active
- 1 cup of bread flour
- 1 cup of flour whole wheat
- ¼ cup of soy flour
- ¼ cup of soymilk powder
- ¼ cup of oat bran
- 1 tbsp of canola oil
- 1 tbsp of honey
- 1 tsp of salt
- 1 cup of water

Directions
In the bread machine pan, arrange the ingredients in an order prescribed by the maker. Choose between the standard medium and regular settings; click Start.

Conclusion

A keto diet may be a healthier option for certain people, although the amount of fat, carbohydrates, and protein prescribed varies from person to person. If you have diabetes, talk to the doctor before starting the diet because it would almost certainly need prescription changes and stronger blood sugar regulation. Are you taking drugs for high blood pressure? Before starting a keto diet again, talk to the doctor. If you're breastfeeding, you shouldn't follow a ketogenic diet. Be mindful that limiting carbs will render you irritable, hungry, and sleepy, among other things. However, this may be a one-time occurrence. Keep in mind that you can eat a balanced diet in order to obtain all of the vitamins and minerals you need. A sufficient amount of fiber is also needed. When the body begins to derive energy from accumulated fat rather than glucose, it is said to be in ketosis. Several trials have shown the powerful weight-loss benefits of a low-carb, or keto, diet. This diet, on the other hand, can be difficult to stick to and can exacerbate health issues in individuals who have certain disorders, such as diabetes type 1. The keto diet is suitable for the majority of citizens. Nonetheless, all major dietary modifications should be discussed with a dietitian or doctor. This is essentially the case with people who have inherent conditions. The keto diet may be an effective therapy for people with drug-resistant epilepsy. Though the diet may be beneficial to people of any age, teenagers, people over 50, and babies can profit the most because they can easily stick to it. Modified keto diets, such as the revised Atkins diet or the low-glycemic index diet, are safer for adolescents and adults. A health care worker should keep a careful eye on someone who is taking a keto diet as a treatment. A doctor and dietitian will maintain track of a person's progress, administer drugs, and test for side effects. The body absorbs fat and protein differently than it does carbohydrates. Carbohydrates have a high insulin reaction. The protein sensitivity to insulin is mild, and the quick insulin response is negligible. Insulin is a fat-producing and fat-conserving enzyme. If you wish to lose weight, consume as many eggs, chickens, fish, and birds as you want, satiate yourself with the fat, and then eat every vegetable that grows on the ground. Butter and coconut oil can be used instead of processed synthetic seed oils. You may be either a sugar or a fat burner, but not both.

www.ingramcontent.com/pod-product-compliance
Lightning Source LLC
Chambersburg PA
CBHW081406080526
44589CB00016B/2481